Ayurvedic Herbal Medicine for Beginners

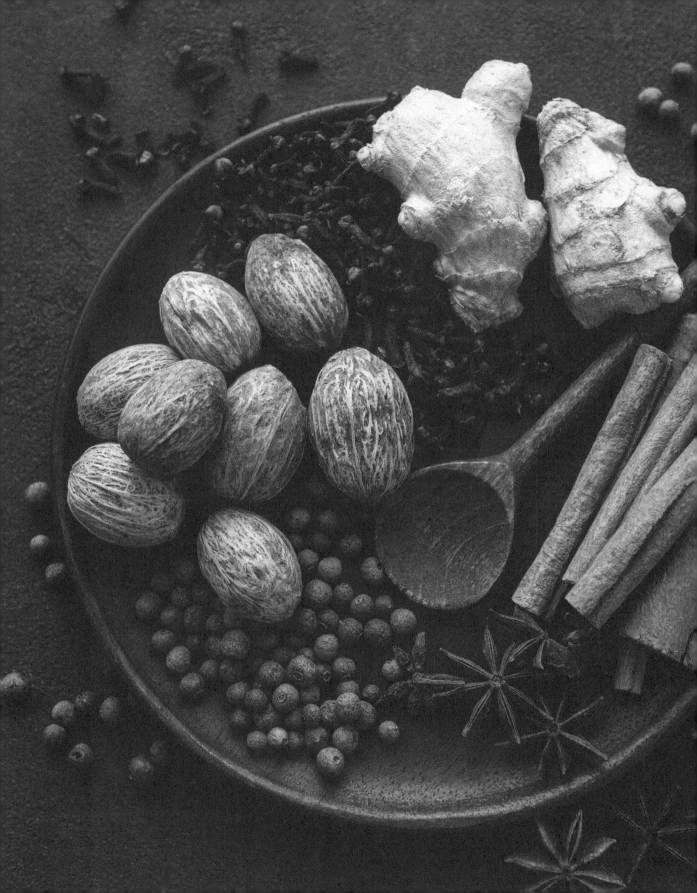

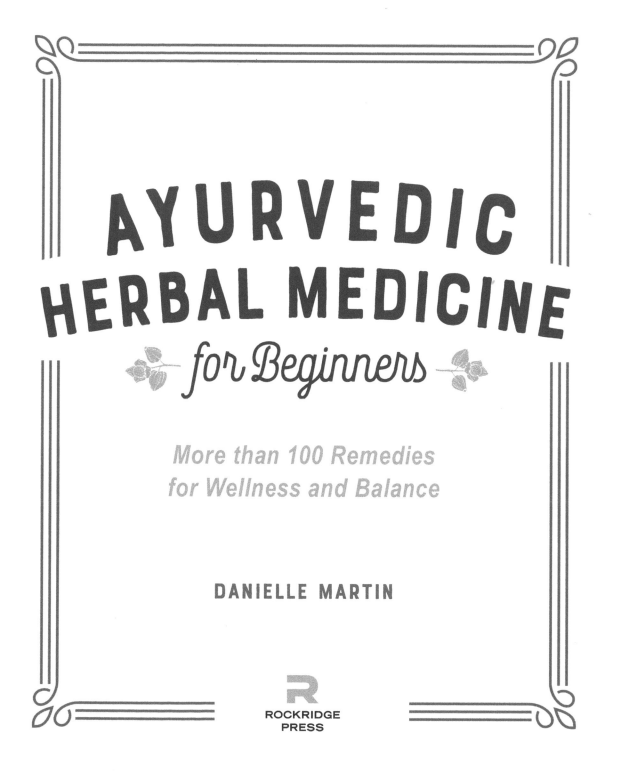

AYURVEDIC HERBAL MEDICINE

for Beginners

More than 100 Remedies
for Wellness and Balance

DANIELLE MARTIN

ROCKRIDGE
PRESS

For my Mom and Pop, who always supported me through my crazy journeys of life, and taught me the greatest gift: to just be me.

For general information on our other products and services or to obtain technical support, please contact our Customer Care Department within the United States at (866) 744-2665, or outside the United States at (510) 253-0500.

Rockridge Press publishes its books in a variety of electronic and print formats. Some content that appears in print may not be available in electronic books, and vice versa.

TRADEMARKS: Rockridge Press and the Rockridge Press logo are trademarks or registered trademarks of Callisto Media Inc. and/or its affiliates, in the United States and other countries, and may not be used without written permission. All other trademarks are the property of their respective owners. Rockridge Press is not associated with any product or vendor mentioned in this book.

Interior and Cover Designer: Gabe Nansen
Art Producer: Janice Ackerman
Editor: Jesse Aylen
Production Editor: Jenna Dutton
Production Manager: Martin Worthington

Alamy: pp. 46, 60, 62, 74, 76, 86, 90, 114, 118; iStock: back cover, ii, pp. 2, 38-39, 40, 70, 84, 88, 106, 116; J. M. Garg: p. 58; Shutterstock: cover, viii-p.1, pp. 8, 16, 22, 30, 48, 50, 52, 54, 56, 64, 66, 68, 72, 78, 80, 82, 92, 94, 96, 98, 100, 102, 104, 108, 110, 112, 190. Author photo courtesy of Jeff Pistana.

Paperback ISBN: 978-1-63807-018-4
eBook ISBN: 978-1-63807-577-6
R0

CONTENTS

INTRODUCTION

Ayurveda is the ancient medical science of India, which uses diet, lifestyle, and herbs to heal imbalance. My journey into Ayurvedic herbology began when I took my first Ayurvedic medicine–making intensive back in 2011 at Alandi Ayurveda Gurukula in Colorado. Although I had already attended a year of Ayurveda school at that point, it was not until this moment that I was able to really delve into the world of Ayurvedic herbology. I was instantly entranced, and from that moment, I spent much of my time making herbal medicines of all kinds for my friends, family, and clients.

Shortly after, I began my first nighantu (an Ayurvedic pharmacopeia) course, which covered more than 100 commonly used Ayurvedic herbs and their energetics, properties, actions, and uses. This in-depth look into Ayurvedic herbalism opened my view to the vast potential that Ayurveda offers and how even simple remedies can bring big changes. Although herbs are just a part of the puzzle, they can truly help heal when used properly.

In the decade since, my herbal medicine practice has evolved greatly. I have created more than 60 Ayurveda-based apothecary products that I sell worldwide. My connection to the herbs has only grown deeper, and I am honored to share a part of this knowledge with you as you begin (or continue) your passage into Ayurvedic medicine.

In the first section of this book, you will find some of the basics of Ayurveda. You will get to know the three doshas (bodily humors), the five elements, the six tastes, the fifteen srotamsi (bodily channels), and the seven dhatus (vital tissues), which collectively set the stage for Ayurvedic herbology. You will also explore your own Ayurvedic constitution, or body type, which will help guide you as you begin to play with the herbal remedies and offerings throughout the book.

The second part takes an in-depth look into 35 commonly used Ayurvedic herbs, their properties, and applications. With this fundamental knowledge, you can begin your journey into home remedies to help conquer numerous day-to-day ailments naturally. The remedies in this book are generally easy and accessible to make, with a wide range of options including teas, honey blends, tinctures, ghees, and oils.

This introduction to Ayurvedic herbalism will provide you with a strong foundation to begin your home herbal practice with great confidence. Although Ayurveda is more than 5,000 years old, as we will explore together, this ancient science can help improve the health and wellness of our society today.

HOW TO USE THIS BOOK

Whether you are a novice or well-established in Ayurveda, this book can hold great value for you. Part 1 sheds light on the fundamentals of Ayurveda. Part 2 offers more tangible information on Ayurvedic herbs that's understandable and easy to incorporate no matter your experience level.

I have gathered this knowledge from invaluable sources, including ancient texts, course notes, personal and clinical experience, and modern books on Ayurvedic medicine. I have condensed and compiled what I believe to be the essence of this knowledge, and my goal is to share it with the highest integrity and utmost gratitude.

As you begin your journey, I recommend you first become acquainted with the various and vital aspects that make Ayurveda so uniquely profound. This includes the three doshas and what they represent, as well as discovering your own dosha type. This is truly foundational knowledge for anyone venturing into the world of Ayurvedic medicine.

Understanding the six tastes will get you more in tune with the herbs, as each taste bestows different properties on its respective herb. By getting to know the srotamsi (bodily channels) and the dhatus (vital tissues) in turn, you will have a deeper understanding of how to use each herb effectively in relation to these parts of the body.

Once you have basic familiarity, you can journey into part 2 and begin to put this information to practical use with recipes and remedies. If you are still scratching your head, take a deep breath and move forward! This book is intended for all levels, so even beginners will be able to grasp the herbal information and remedies with confidence.

Overall, you'll become familiar with these 35 Ayurvedic herbs, their specific actions and properties, and how you can use them in your day-to-day life for many common ailments like cough, cold, insomnia, anxiety, digestion issues, weight issues, and toxicity. I'll also share some simple remedies for alleviating these ailments in the comfort of your home.

Although this is a book on herbal medicine, Ayurveda goes way beyond that realm. Ayurveda is total life medicine, and without addressing necessary factors in your diet and lifestyle, the herbal remedies will go only so far. Nonetheless, herbs are Mother Nature's treasures, which can complement any well-rounded health-care plan for quicker, more encompassing, and more powerful results.

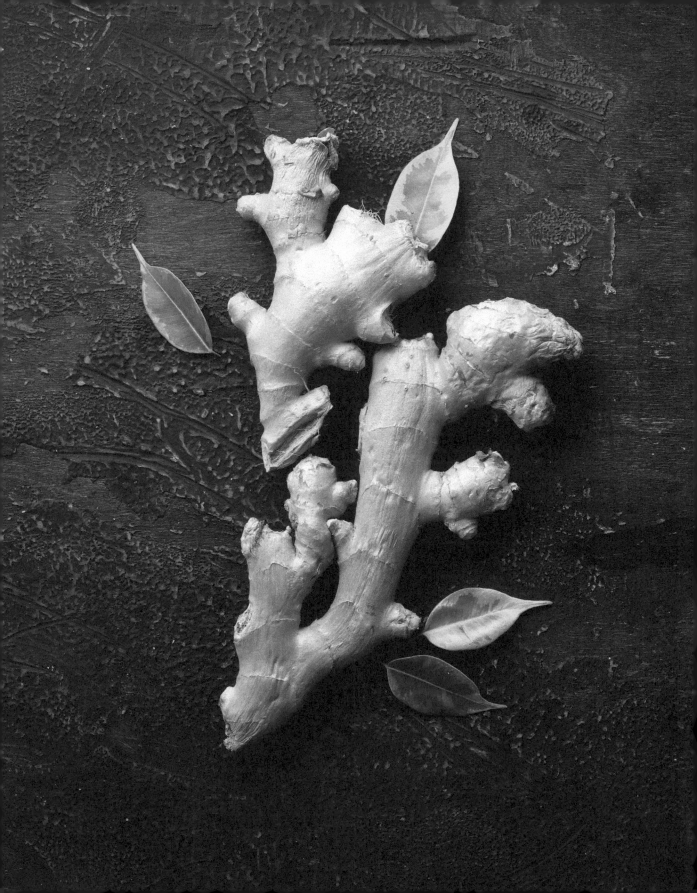

PART ONE

AYURVEDA BASICS

In this section, we will establish the basics of Ayurveda and how they relate to herbal medicine. You will learn about the Vata, Pitta, and Kapha doshas, the five elements from which they come, and how they manifest in your body. We will touch on the concepts of rasa (taste), virya (potency), vipak (post-digestive), and prabhava (special property) and why they are essential components of Ayurvedic medicine. Through this foundational knowledge, you can begin to deepen your herbal practice and use the remedies to their fullest potential.

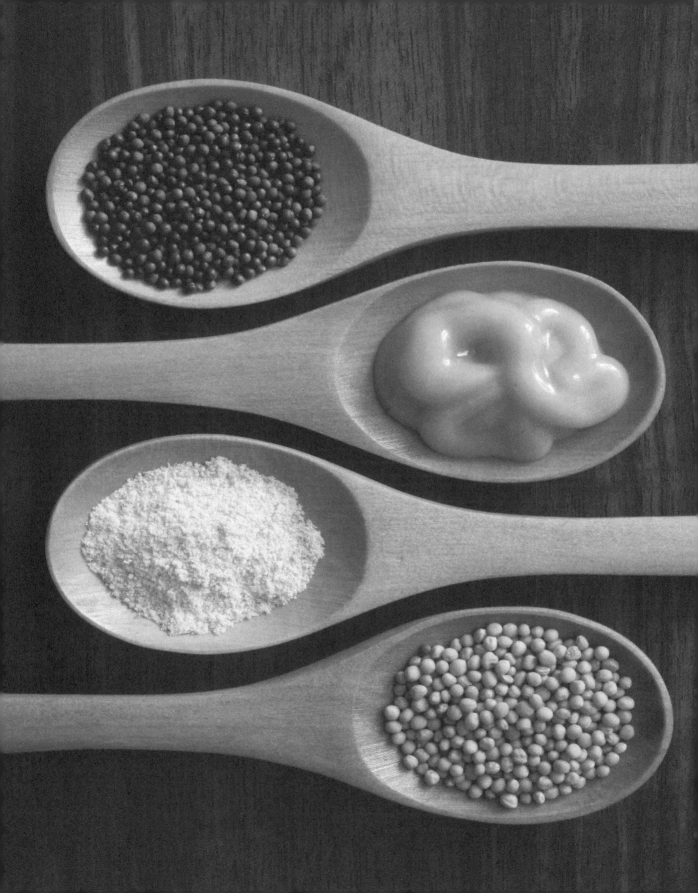

Chapter One

AYURVEDA 101

Let us begin this journey by looking into Ayurveda's origins. Since Ayurveda is a spiritual science, it is important to honor its roots and maintain its original integrity, so that we can keep its torch burning.

Ayurveda may be more than 5,000 years old, but it holds great relevance in our modern society and has helped to shape many aspects of modern medicine and Western herbalism today. In fact, with its personalized approach and adaptable guidelines, Ayurveda is more needed than ever. Ayurveda is considered a "living" science, meaning it is not a fixed set of concepts but can easily be modified and individualized to fit everyone's unique needs.

Before we venture too deeply into the herbal medicine component, let's talk about how to use this information safely and how to sustainably source the herbs we will discuss in part 2.

ORIGINS OF AYURVEDA

Ayurveda is an ancient medical system that originated in India thousands of years ago. In the beginning, Ayurveda was strictly an oral tradition—in other words, one that was passed down verbally—making its precise origin difficult to establish. Many claim Ayurveda began around the 2nd century BCE, although it is thought by some to be much older.

According to Hindu mythology, Ayurveda was created by Lord Brahma—fittingly, the Lord of Creation. It was then passed on to several other Hindu gods, including Lord Daksha Prajapati (son of Brahma), Lord Indra (king of the gods), the Ashwini twins (physicians of the gods), and Lord Dhanvantari (father of Ayurveda; the first divine incarnation to impart Ayurveda to humankind). It was revealed to the ancient rishis (saints) of India here on earth through deep meditation, then passed on to their devoted students.

The first documentation of Ayurveda is found in the Atharva Veda, one of the four sacred ancient Hindu scriptures (1200 BCE–1000 BCE), which talks about spells, rituals, and procedures of daily life. It was the first Indian text to discuss medicine and disease classification, and it identifies plant-based medicine in its hymns and verses.

Many years after the Atharva Veda was compiled, several other great texts were written by the ancient vaidyas (doctors) and their disciples. The three most well-known, Caraka Samhita, Sushruta Samhita, and Ashtanga Hridayam, make up the Bruhat Trayi, or "three greats," of Ayurveda.

The science of Ayurveda is based on the Shad Darshanas, the six systems of Indian philosophy. Although these systems vary in their methods and ideology, their purpose remains constant: to eliminate worldly suffering through the realization of the true Self. Hence, Ayurveda has been created to end the physical and mental suffering that is common in us all.

Ayurveda is a well-rounded system of medicine comprising eight branches or limbs, including Kaya Chikitsa (internal medicine), Bala Chikitsa (pediatrics), Graha Chikitsa (demonology and psychology), Shalakya Tantra (ear, nose, and throat), Shalya Tantra (surgery), Agad Tantra (toxicology), Jara-Rasayana Chikitsa (geriatrics and rejuvenation), and Vajikarana Chikitsa (aphrodisiac therapy).

One profound, eternal aspect of Ayurveda is its definition of perfect health, or svastha. Unlike Western medicine, Ayurveda claims that health is not merely the absence of disease. For perfect health, one must have balanced doshas (Vata, Pitta, Kapha), dhatus (vital tissues), agni (digestion), mala (excreta), manas (mind), and indriya (senses).

Ayurveda Now

Although Ayurveda is fundamentally rooted in India, you can come to it from any background, age, race, ethnicity, gender, identity, religion, or dietary preference. It is graciously all-inclusive! As Ayurveda continues to grow in popularity in the West, many Ayurvedic products are sold online and in general health-food stores, and Ayurvedic clinics, spas, and schools are now opening throughout North America and Europe. Whether you are from the East or West, Ayurveda can help you on your health and wellness journey.

Ayurveda aims to balance the body, mind, and consciousness of each individual through the holistic measures of diet, lifestyle, and herbs. As a living science, it is extremely adaptable and its principles are applicable to modern health-care needs, especially in today's overly prescribed society. Ayurveda takes each individual's personal needs into consideration and does not offer one-size-fits-all remedies or demand an "all-or-nothing" way of life. Start small! The practical, accessible home remedies in this book offer many options to find balance naturally. Once you have gained a more thorough understanding of the subtypes of Vata, the three doshas, and engaged with the rest of the foundational knowledge in this chapter and the following ones, you will be equipped to adapt Ayurveda's many healing properties to your own life as best suits you.

Understanding the Five Subtypes of Vata

Composed of Air and Ether, Vata dosha is the biological, energetic force that controls all movement in the body, including respiration, circulation, and digestion. The five subtypes of Vata, or five Vayus (winds), hold great significance in Ayurvedic medicine and in our health.

Prana Vayu lives in the mind and heart. Prana flows down and inward, and it governs our inhalation. Healthy Prana is necessary for proper attention, perception, thinking, and feeling. Many emotional-mental disorders are rooted in this wind.

Udana Vayu lives in the diaphragm, lungs, and throat, and this energy flows upward. Udana controls our exhalations and stimulates speech, memory, enthusiasm, and self-will.

Vyana Vayu lives in the heart and flows through the bloodstream. Vyana helps deliver nutrients and oxygen to all our vital tissues, maintains healthy circulation, and controls cardiac functioning.

Samana Vayu lives in the small intestines and navel region; as a meeting point of Prana and Apana, it is a "balancing wind." This wind plays an important role in digestion, absorption, and assimilation; many digestive disorders involve an imbalance in Samana.

Apana Vayu lives in the colon and pelvic cavity; it moves in a down-and-out direction. As the downward wind, Apana is responsible for bowel movements, urination, menstruation, and childbirth. Healthy Apana grounds our energy and emotions.

SAFETY RECOMMENDATIONS

There are many factors to consider for safe usage of the herbs in Ayurveda. Every herb has a list of precautions, or instances when it should be avoided. These are listed with each individual herb and should be carefully noted and applied.

Some medications can cause unwanted drug-herb interactions. Likewise, some herbs can block the effective component of a drug or increase its absorbency. When an herb and drug have similar actions (e.g., if both lower blood sugar), close monitoring from your doctor will be required to see if the medication needs to be adjusted. You can find some useful websites that offer comprehensive lists of drug-herb interactions in the Resources section on page 195.

Before using the herbs, talk with your doctor if you are currently on medications, experiencing any serious illness, or are pregnant or breastfeeding. These remedies are not meant to replace any medical advice from your physician. Your doctor can help to assess whether a chosen remedy is appropriate given any other treatments you may be concurrently taking or undergoing.

SOURCING HERBS

Some of the herbs in these pages may be new to you. Before purchasing any herbs, it is important to know where they are coming from. Ayurvedic herbs have been linked to heavy metal toxicity, making it extremely vital to source your herbs from a trusted supplier. Sadly, just because an herb is labeled organic does not ensure it is free from heavy metals.

Sustainability is another important factor to consider when sourcing your herbs. Many herbs are classified as endangered, often due to irresponsible overharvesting methods. Do your part to keep our herbs safe and make sure your herbal retailer sources strictly from sustainable farming and harvesting suppliers.

See the Resources section on page 195 for some herbal companies that supply clean and sustainably grown herbs and products. These companies can help ensure that you are practicing Ayurvedic herbal medicine in a responsible and ethical fashion with their thoughtful and sustainable harvesting methodologies.

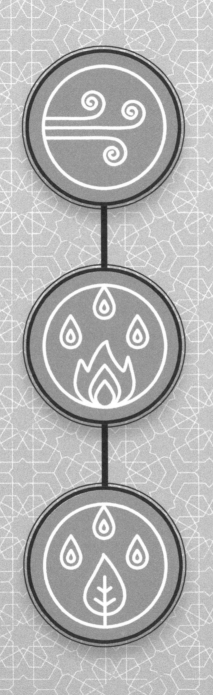

Chapter Two

CONSTITUTIONAL TYPES AND THE THREE DOSHAS

If you are new to the concept of the doshas, they may appear abstract at first because they're formless and energy-based. Nonetheless, the doshic paradigm is a unique and invaluable component of Ayurveda. Understanding it is key to utilizing Ayurveda's fullest potential.

A *dosha* is a Sanskrit term that is often translated as "bodily humor." It's a subtle, energetic, biological force that governs our actions, physical characteristics, personalities, and mental-emotional dispositions. The three doshas are Vata, Pitta, and Kapha. Each dosha is made from two of the five elements (Ether, Air, Fire, Water, and Earth) and expresses the qualities that reflect the attributes of those elements.

We each carry all three doshas in our system, but the ratio in which they show up makes up our Prakriti (individual constitution) and serves as the blueprint for our physical and mental traits.

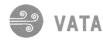 **VATA**

Vata dosha is born from Air and Ether. Its main qualities include rough, light, cold, hard, coarse, non-slimy (dry), mobile, and clear. Although Vata travels throughout the body, its "home base" is in the colon; hence, the first symptoms of elevated Vata often show up in this region (e.g., gas, bloating, constipation). Vata also tends to accumulate in the head, mind, nervous system, heart, throat, diaphragm, small intestine, pelvic cavity, lower back, bones, and thighs. For example, high Vata may lead to anxiety (mind), osteoporosis (bones), heart palpitations (heart), or sciatica (lower back).

Vata's main functions include respiration, circulation, perception, sensation, digestion, and elimination. Strong and healthy Vata is needed for proper performance of these vital tasks, while imbalanced Vata creates trouble or affliction in these areas. Balanced Vata maintains proper activity of everything in our system; an imbalance will lead to stagnation, pain, and disharmony.

Individuals who are predominant in Vata will often share the same qualities of this dosha. Common characteristics include being underweight, fragile, quick, anxious, and imaginative. These individuals are often highly sensitive and may be affected easily by energy, scents, and noises. A healthy Vata type is often adaptable, creative, silly, talkative, and rarely boring. They are abundant with amazing ideas, but their creative potential is often unfulfilled due to a lack of focus. Vata types are generally active, restless, and crave change, even though a stable routine is one of their best medicines. When imbalanced, a Vata type may be prone to anxiety, insomnia, constipation, gas, bloating, dryness, hypersensitivity, and hyperactivity.

Sensitive Vata types may be exceptionally responsive to the effects of herbs. It may be wise to start with a lower dose of an herb and increase slowly, if appropriate. In general, Vata does well with unctuous (oily), heavy herbs of a sweet nature such as Bala and Yashtimadhu (licorice), as well as herbs that have a direct affinity for the nervous system such as Ashwagandha and Shankapushpi. Herbs that have a strong bitter or astringent taste are often too cooling, cleansing, and drying for Vata.

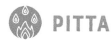 **PITTA**

Pitta dosha comprises Fire and Water and is naturally hot, sharp (penetrating), spreading, oily, light, and liquid in quality. The word *Pitta* comes from the word "tap," meaning heat, as well as austerity (both of which are powerful attributes of Pitta). Pitta plays a large role in digestion and lives in the lower stomach and small intestine. Pitta disorders may show up as inflammation, heat, burning, or acidity in the gut (e.g., celiac disease, Crohn's disease, ulcer, hyperacidity). Other main sites include the liver, skin, mind, eyes, blood, and navel region; these areas often attract Pitta disorders. For instance, excessive Pitta in the mind will lead to anger, frustration, and judgment, and elevated Pitta in the skin (and liver) may manifest as acne, eczema, dermatitis, or rashes.

Pitta governs transformation. It is responsible for turning food into absorbable nutrients and thoughts into feelings and emotions. Without healthy Pitta, neither your food nor your thoughts will be processed properly, and physical and mental toxins can emerge. Alternatively, a strong, balanced Pitta can digest even the heaviest of foods and emotions without hesitation.

Pitta-predominant individuals are generally focused, driven, and sharp-minded. They are often prestigious. They have set goals and the discipline to accomplish them. Physically, they tend toward average height, medium weight; warm, flushed skin; fine hair (with premature hair loss and graying), and medium, almond-shaped eyes. When Pitta is elevated, a person may become egotistical, overly critical, and judgmental. Their ambition and perfectionist nature may steer them toward obsession, overwork, and burnout. Nonetheless, Pitta types are extremely loyal, honest, motivational, and hold great potential.

Because Pitta has a strong constitution and strong digestion, these individuals often process herbs quite well. However, their hot nature can easily become provoked, and heating herbs such as Chitrak, Maricha (black pepper), and Shunti (dry ginger) should be avoided or used sparingly. In contrast, Pitta finds cooling herbs such as Shatavari and Yashtimadhu quite soothing. Bitter is also better with Pitta; it's not only cooling, but often acts directly on the liver, making herbs such as Kutki and Neem common Pitta favorites.

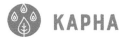 **KAPHA**

Kapha dosha comes from Water and Earth. Its qualities are heavy, dull, slow, cool, oily, hard, dense, soft, liquid, and gross. This dosha is our "building block" and makes up most of our bodily structures, from the tiniest cells to our tissues, organs, and systems. Kapha's main residence is in the upper stomach (fundus), and an initial increase in Kapha may show up as dull appetite, an undue feeling of fullness, sluggish digestion, nausea, or sleepiness after food. Kapha also resides in the lungs, joints, saliva, mind, plasma, lymphatic tissue, pancreas, cerebrospinal fluid, and sinus cavity. If Kapha increases, it may affect these areas, resulting in a dull or foggy mind, excessive mucus, thick saliva, lymphatic congestion, or insulin resistance.

Kapha is responsible for lubrication and supports our bodies and minds. Healthy Kapha provides strength, stamina, growth, immunity, and vitality. Kapha grounds us and sets the stage for relaxation and deep sleep when balanced. Given its soft, oily nature, Kapha also provides love, compassion, and contentment.

A Kapha individual may be loving, caring, affectionate, and nurturing. They are often easygoing and agreeable, and they do not like conflict. Their go-with-the-flow attitude and strong loyalty can sometimes make them better followers than leaders. Due to their watery nature, they can be very emotional and may cry often and easily (even when happy). Physically, Kapha types often have a large, strong, solid body frame; big, beautiful eyes; youthful, glowing skin; thick, healthy hair; and a melodious voice. When Kapha is increased, weight gain, slow metabolism, congestion, brain fog, sluggishness, and low motivation may result.

Kapha types are strong and sturdy and can generally handle herbs in generous amounts. With their heavy, slow, and oily nature, Kapha individuals tend to do best with herbs that are light, stimulating, and drying, such as Punarnava, Chitrak, and Shunti (dry ginger), which help kindle digestion and metabolism. Herbs of a heavy, sweet, and starchy nature should be avoided, however, as these qualities will likely lead to congestion, heaviness, and toxicity.

Discovering Ayurvedic Herbs

Ayurvedic herbalism evolved from thousands of years of clinical trial, observation, and experience. Through these efforts, we have a map of each herb, their qualities (guna), and their actions (karma). Each herb exhibits specific tastes (rasa), heating or cooling energy (virya), and post-digestive effect (vipak), revealing their health properties, when to use them, and when to avoid them.

One of Ayurveda's greatest acknowledgments is the fact that we are all unique beings with unique needs. It is essential to remember this when using herbs as well; A does not always equal B, and what heals one person may be harmful to another. For example, Chitrak is excellent for increasing digestion, but if there is inflammation and acidity in the gastrointestinal tract, this heating herb will worsen the condition. Alternatively, Chitrak can be used for a dull appetite and sluggish metabolism with great results.

As you continue reading, you will learn about the fundamentals of Ayurvedic herbalism and why they are so vital when choosing and using your herbs. You will also see notations throughout speaking to the balances of rasa, virya, and vipak for each remedy. By getting to know the herbs this way, you can begin to use them safely, effectively, and to their greatest potential.

In the next couple of pages, you will have the chance to assess yourself through the understanding of your doshas. We will accomplish this by using a straightforward quiz that delves more intentionally into personal characteristics and how they align with each dosha in turn.

Discover Your Dosha (Constitution) Type

Now that you understand a little about each dosha, let's explore how they relate to your own personal characteristics. By knowing which dosha(s) is/are predominant in your constitution, you can determine which herbs to favor and which ones to avoid. Although these quizzes have their limitations, this is a helpful first step on the path to personal balance. Evaluate your own individual situation for each characteristic by reading through each of these categories and assessing which ones most align to yourself. Then keep these findings in mind, particularly the balance between Vata, Pitta, and Kapha, as you embark upon using the herbs and remedies.

CHARACTERISTIC	VATA	PITTA	KAPHA
BODY FRAME	Small Fragile Thin	Medium Medium strength Average	Large Strong Solid
BODY WEIGHT	Underweight	Average	Overweight
SKIN TYPE	Dry Scaly Flaky or wrinkled	Flushed Fair Oily	Cool Clammy Clear, soft, or wrinkle-free
EYES	Small Beady Dry	Medium Penetrating Itchy or irritated	Large Beautiful Watery
HAIR	Coarse Frizzy Dry	Fine Straight Prematurely gray Thinning	Thick Lustrous Oily
APPETITE	Irregular Forgets to eat Spacey hunger	Strong Never misses a meal Cranky hunger	Dull Skips meals easily No hunger
DIGESTION	Gas Bloating Sensitive to raw food and proteins	Hyperacidity Inflammation Sensitive to spicy and oily foods	Slow Sluggish Sensitive to dairy, gluten, and grains

CHARACTERISTIC	VATA	PITTA	KAPHA
ELIMINATION	Dry stools Constipation Skips days	Loose stools Overactive 3+ daily	Balanced Well-formed 1 or 2 daily
CIRCULATION & TEMPERATURE	Poor circulation Cold Modest sweat	Strong circulation Hot Medium-high sweat Strong scent	Poor circulation Cool Clammy Excessive sweat
SLEEP	Poor Light	Medium Balanced or Average	Heavy Excessive
CLIMATE PREFERENCE	Hot High humidity	Cold Moderate humidity	Warm Low to no humidity
EMOTIONAL TENDENCIES	Anxiety Fear Worry Grief Fluctuating	Anger Irritation Impatience Intense	Sadness Depression Grief Surpressed
MIND & INTELLECT	Spacy Restless Overactive Forgetful Creative	Sharp, witty Perfectionist Focused Strong memory Debater	Dull Foggy Slow thinker Dislikes debate Goes with flow
WORK HABITS	Irregular Changes jobs often Lacks focus Active work	Motivated Self-driven Workaholic Critical thinking Entrepreneur	Loyal worker Slow and steady Poor motivation Sedentary work
TEMPERAMENT	Active Talkative Silly Changeable	Serious Passionate Charismatic Motivational	Mellow Patient Nurturing Compassionate Loving

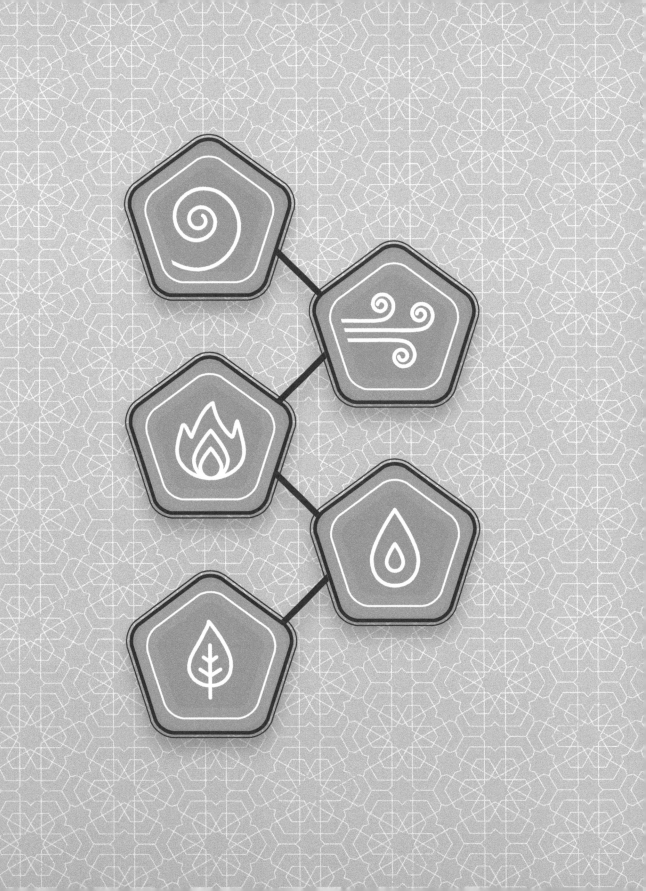

Chapter Three

FIVE ELEMENTS OF AYURVEDA

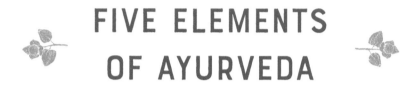

Ayurveda is based on a theory of evolution as humans having transformed from a state of unmanifest (meaning "nothingness") to the manifested world of material creation. From this, the five great elements, or Pancha Mahabhutas, arose, bringing us the balancing elements of Ether, Air, Fire, Water, and Earth.

In Ayurveda, all organic and inorganic matter contains all five elements—the building blocks of creation. However, their ratios vary, and this determines the unique qualities of any given substance, be it a human being, animal, plant, food, or rock.

Ayurvedic herbalism is intimately connected to the five elements. Each herb represents the chief elements it comes from, determining its properties, uses, and indications, which guide us when it is best and most ideal to use them. By knowing the predominant elements of each herb, we can decipher the best herbs to bring us balance.

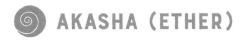

AKASHA (ETHER)

Akasha (Ether) is the first of the five great elements, as everything is born out of space. It is all-pervasive and omnipresent. The qualities of space include clear, subtle, light, infinite, and eternal. Because it is one of the main elements of Vata dosha, Vata shares many of these qualities as well.

Akasha relates to the ears and sense of hearing, as sound needs space to travel. It was within the eternal space that the first primordial sound of AUM was created, giving rise to the physical universe. Space is necessary for freedom, love, acceptance, and receptivity, making it a beautiful element to carry in our daily lives. However, excessive Akasha can lead to spaciness, forgetfulness, and lack of grounding.

In plants, Akasha manifests as the fruit, which holds its essence and means to procreate. Herbs that are light and subtle may be predominant in Ether and can be helpful in times of too much heaviness. This can be seen with herbs such as Kutki, Neem, and Kalmegha.

VAYU (AIR)

From Akasha, movement arose to form Air, or Vayu (wind). Without wind, no life is possible. Prana (the life force) is the essence of wind and governs all movement, in ourselves and in the universe. The qualities of wind include mobile, light, clear, dry, rough, and unstable. Vayu is responsible for respiration, circulation, digestion, and elimination.

Vayu relates to the skin and sense of touch (as a breeze felt against the skin, for example). It also governs the nervous system; its movement allows electrical impulses to exist. Vayu keeps our systems flowing freely, so stagnation can lead to pain and inflammation. Healthy Vayu creates positive action, adaptability, and energy. Meanwhile, excessive Vayu leads to restlessness, hyperactivity, sleeplessness, lack of focus, and lack of direction.

In plants, Vayu is found in the leaves, the location of veins and vascular tissue. Herbs with a strong Vayu presence are light, drying, and stimulating, and are useful when dealing with lethargy, sluggish digestion, congestion, and poor circulation. Notable Vayu herbs include Maricha (black pepper), Shunti (dry ginger), and Neem.

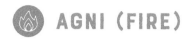 AGNI (FIRE)

From Air, friction occurred and created Agni, the fire element. Agni, or Tejas, is our transformational potential, processing all things. Fire's characteristics include hot, sharp, penetrating, spreading, illuminating, and light. Agni is responsible for digestion, comprehension, and intelligence. Because Pitta has a strong Fire influence, this dosha shares many similar attributes.

Agni is connected to the eyes and sense of sight, which gives birth to form. The fire element is also required for thinking, perceiving, processing, and digesting. It turns thought into knowledge and feelings and turns food into absorbable nutrients. A strong Agni bestows focus, ambition, and drive, and maintains bodily temperature and a radiant complexion. An overactive fire invokes inflammation, irritation, anger, criticism, and obsession.

In plants, Agni is found in the flower, with its beautiful color and form. Its luminosity attracts creatures of all kinds. An herb with a strong Agni component will be heating, penetrating, and drying. This can be observed with herbs such as Chitrak, Maricha (black pepper), and Sarshapa (brown mustard seed).

APAS (WATER)

From fire, condensation was born to create the Water element, or Apas (also Ap or Jala). Water is vital for life on Earth. Our human bodies are more than 60 percent water, and Earth's surface is 70 percent water. Without water, life could not exist. Water is cool, fluid, heavy, soft, dull, slow, and slimy. Besides sustaining life, water is necessary for assimilating nutrients, hydration, and cohesion. Because Kapha is born from Apas, many of its qualities are the same.

Water is connected with the tongue and sense of taste, because taste is not possible if your mouth is completely dry. Healthy Apas and proper hydration are necessary for cleansing and maintaining nutrition and lymphatic health. A strong Apas promotes fluidity, softness, love, affection, and compassion. Excessive water can lead to retention, swelling, congestion, attachment, and an overflow of emotions.

Apas is connected to the stem of the plant, the pathway of its water source and nutrition. Water-predominant herbs are often oily, moisturizing, and soothing. Such herbs include Yashtimadhu (licorice) and Shatavari.

PRITHVI (EARTH)

Minerals from Water soon solidified to form the solid Earth, known as Prithvi. In the universe, Earth provides us with home, food, and shelter. It is our temple and greatest healer. In our bodies, Prithvi bestows grounding, relaxation, and deep sleep. Prithvi is the building block of all material structures in the universe and in our bodies. Prithvi is heavy, gross, stable, dense, hard, dull, and slow, and is a strong component of Kapha.

Prithvi is connected to the nose and sense of smell. Earth and its minerals exude a powerful scent. Healthy Prithvi is essential for staying centered and calm and for warding off restlessness, hyperactivity, and sleeplessness. Too much Earth can lead to sluggish digestion, weight gain, lethargy, dull mind, and depression.

In plants, Prithvi is found in the roots, due to their close connection to Mother Earth. Herbs with a strong Prithvi component are dense, heavy, and calming and possess a strong scent, as with Ashwagandha.

The Elements and Your Ayurvedic Practice

We are made up of all five elements, but some are more pronounced than others. By identifying the main elements in your constitution, you can begin to decode your own personal diet, lifestyle, and herbal needs.

Opposites tend to balance each other out, so if you have one or more overactive elements in your constitution, you will likely need to favor opposite elements to find balance. Ether and Air can be calmed by Earth and Water, Fire can be soothed by Water and Earth, and Water and Earth can avoid stagnation with Ether, Air, and Fire.

Because each dosha relates to two of the elements, you can often determine your dominant elements by learning your dosha type. This reveals what foods or herbs may be healing for you and which ones may lead to imbalance. For instance, if you are a Kapha type, you will likely have strong Earth and Water elements in your system. By adopting food, activities, and herbs with strong Ether, Air, and Fire components, you can keep your mind sharp and clear and your body light and energized.

Discovering Ayurvedic Herbs: Rasayana

Ayurveda offers many different therapeutic classifications that indicate each herb's qualities and uses. One of the main categories is Rasayana (rejuvenation) herbs. Although Rasayana herbs can be used for many purposes, they are often administered after a cleanse or illness or any time there is weakness and depletion.

Although there are exceptions, Rasayana herbs are often heavy, starchy, moisturizing, and nourishing. They are tonics, meaning that they strengthen and tone the body by building tissue and providing nutrition. They are considered antiaging and promote strength, energy, and longevity.

Before using these building herbs, it is important to know that due to their heavy, oily qualities, many Rasayana herbs will provoke congestion and toxicity if toxins are already present. They can be hard to digest, and if the Agni (digestive fire) is low, these starchy herbs will further clog the system. Therefore, keep your digestion robust and your system cleansed before taking these nourishing tonics in abundance.

There are countless Rasayana herbs available. Some classic examples include Ashwagandha, Shatavari, and Bala. However, some more surprising rejuvenative herbs include Neem, Chitrak, and Pippali.

The next chapter will provide a deeper look into the facets of Ayurveda along with the Six Tastes common throughout Ayurvedic healing and remedies.

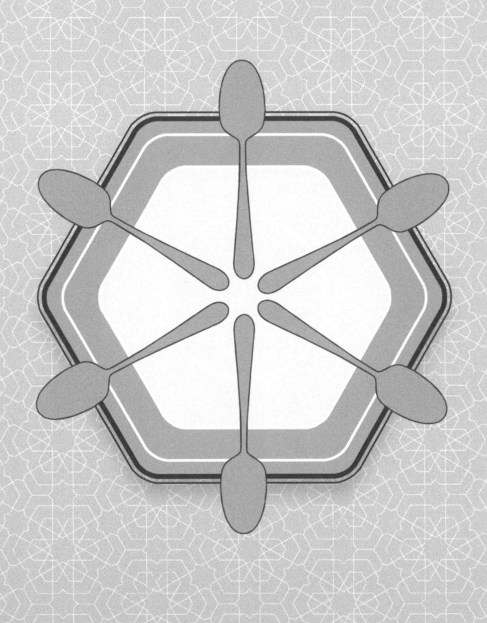

Chapter Four

RASA, VIRYA, VIPAK, PRABHAVA, AND THE SIX TASTES

The concepts of rasa (taste), virya (potency), vipak (post-digestive effect), and prabhava (specific action) are profoundly important within Ayurveda. Without some knowledge of these herbal fundamentals, true Ayurvedic herbalism is not possible. In this chapter, we will cover the definitions of these abstractions and why they are an essential part of Ayurvedic medicine. You will begin to understand the subtle aspects of each herb in order to determine the best times for use, when to avoid them, and how to combine them for greater balance.

Ayurveda talks a great deal about the six tastes. Each taste arises from two elements and affects the doshas, digestion, body, and mind accordingly. The taste an herb exhibits also corresponds to its healing potential, therapeutic uses, potency (i.e., heating or cooling), and potential precautions. No other system of medicine acknowledges this method of exploration, yet Ayurvedic herbalism is incomplete without it. Keep reading to discover the six tastes, their corresponding elements, and their effects on our systems.

RASA (TASTE)

Rasa has many translations, including "essence," "juice," and "taste." Rasa denotes the taste of an herb but also represents its essence. The rasa occurs in the mouth and is a critical part of the digestion process. To digest and absorb the herbs, it is important to take them in a form that allows you to fully taste them, rather than swallow them in the form of a capsule or pill.

There are six different rasas: madhura (sweet), amla (sour), lavana (saline), katu (pungent), tikta (bitter), and kashaya (astringent), each of which possesses its own unique attributes and effects. Knowing the rasa of an herb will give you an idea of its subsequent virya (potency) and vipak (post-digestive effect), as well as its actions on the doshas, dhatus (tissues), and malas (waste products).

VIRYA (POTENCY)

Virya is often translated as "energy" or "potency." There are eight types; however, for simplicity, virya is commonly referred to by two types: ushna (heating) and shita (cooling). The virya's effect tends to overpower the rasa in herbal medicine. In fact, the Caraka Samhita, a Sanskrit Ayurvedic book, boldly states that "the virya is responsible for each and every action." The virya acts in the stomach and small intestines and directly affects Agni (digestive fire).

Generally speaking, cooling herbs are anabolic (building), moisturizing, nourishing, and rejuvenating. They tend to reduce heat and pacify Pitta but aggravate both Vata and Kapha. Alternatively, heating herbs are catabolic (reducing), drying, and digestive. They increase sweating, thirst, body temperature, and circulation. Heating herbs often reduce Kapha and Vata and provoke Pitta.

VIPAK (POST-DIGESTIVE EFFECT)

Vipak, the post-digestive effect, prevails over the rasa and virya of an herb (although all are important). It is the final, most subtle, and longest-acting stage. Vipak lives in the colon; its effects are felt in the malas (excreta) and dhatus (tissues) after digestion.

Vipak relates to the tastes and is labeled as madhura (sweet), amla (sour), or katu (pungent). Because we cannot taste the herbs during this stage, they have been classified by their actions on the body. A sweet vipak is oily and heavy, increases Kapha, and promotes energy, semen, and elimination. A sour vipak is oily and light, aggravates Pitta, and promotes appetite, digestion, and elimination. A pungent vipak is dry and light, disturbs Vata (and sometimes Pitta), and is reducing and constricting (constipative).

PRABHAVA (SPECIFIC ACTION)

Although we have explored the general rules of rasa, virya, and vipak, there are countless exceptions. When an herb exhibits a certain rasa, virya, and vipak yet has a completely different, unexpected effect on the body, this is known as prabhava. Prabhava is the unexplainable action an herb carries, despite all logical reasoning.

As you go through the herbal directory, you may begin to pick up on these abnormalities. For instance, Guduchi is heating, yet it is one of the best herbs for treating Pitta. Kalmegha is one of the most bitter herbs (which are generally cooling), yet it is extremely heating. Although most powdered herbs have a one-year shelf life, Vidanga, Pippali, and Dhanya (coriander) actually increase in potency with age.

THE SIX TASTES

Now that we've discussed the six tastes and their great importance, let us uncover their unique attributes and specific actions, and how they relate to herbalism.

Sweet—Water and Earth

Madhura, or the sweet taste, is composed of Water and Earth and has affinity for the thyroid gland. It is cooling, anabolic, and heavy. It reduces Vata and Pitta but increases Kapha.

Madhura nourishes all seven dhatus (vital tissues); bolsters strength, rejuvenation, and libido; encourages healthy elimination; and supports graceful aging. When used properly, the sweet taste promotes love, compassion, contentment, and satisfaction. Excessive madhura leads to attachment, greed, lethargy, obesity, sluggish digestion, hypothyroidism, goiter, tumors, and metabolic disorders.

Many Rasayana (rejuvenative) herbs bestow a sweet taste, including Ashwagandha, Bala, and Shatavari. These herbs are beneficial during times of low energy, depletion, and Vata imbalance but should be avoided with toxins, congestion, or Kapha provocation.

Many aromatic spices are enticingly sweet, as you will find with Tvak (cinnamon), Ela (cardamom), Mishreya (fennel), Ardraka (fresh ginger), and Dhanya (coriander). Their pleasing aromas will spark your Agni (digestion) and your appetite.

Sour—Fire and Earth

Sour is known as *amla* in Ayurveda and comes from Fire and Earth. Amla has an affinity for the lungs and is heating, anabolic, and unctuous by nature. It reduces Vata but aggravates Pitta. Amla initially decreases Kapha but will provoke it with excessive use.

The sour taste promotes salivation, stimulates digestion and metabolism, and alleviates symptoms of dypepsia, such as gas and bloating. In healthy amounts, amla awakens the mind and energizes the body. It supports satisfaction and discernment. In excess, amla can lead to criticism, resentfulness, hyperacidity, ulceration, inflammation, thirst, and congestion, as well as skin disorders.

Many herbs that contain the sour taste are also high in vitamin C, making them powerful antioxidants, immune boosters, and liver tonics. Quite possibly, the most well-known sour herb in Ayurveda is Amalaki, whose name itself means "sour."

Salty—Fire and Water

Lavana, or salt, is the taste ruled by Fire and Water. Lavana is heating, metabolic, and oily in its properties. Due to its association with Water, salt has affinity for the kidneys. Lavana alleviates Vata but will increase Pitta and Kapha.

The salty taste restores appetite, improves digestion, enhances flavor, promotes elimination (laxative), relieves gas, cleanses, softens, and moisturizes. It provides energy, inspiration, confidence, and enthusiasm. Lack of salty taste can lead to dullness and boredom. When taken in excess, lavana gives rise to heat, thirst, inflammation, ulceration, acidity, water retention, hypertension, skin disorders, impotency, wrinkles, gray hair, hair loss, attachment, greed, and addiction.

Although not many herbs are salty, you can get a subtle taste with Shilajit, a mineral-rich, tar-like resin. Of course, the most powerful way to obtain the salt taste is through salt itself, with pink Himalayan salt being the best option—it is less heating, less provoking to the doshas, and lower in sodium than other salts.

Pungent—Fire and Air

Pungent (spicy) is known as *katu* and is made of Fire and Air. It has an affinity for the heart and stomach and is heating, drying, lightening, and metabolic. Because of this, katu increases Pitta and alleviates Kapha. A small amount will warm up Vata, but overuse will deplete and dry out this dosha.

Katu stimulates digestion, absorption, metabolism, and circulation. It is naturally cleansing, antiparasitical, and antimicrobial. Katu clears the senses, thins the blood, removes congestion, and reduces fat. It improves clarity, focus, and intellect. With overconsumption, however, katu leads to heat, inflammation, anger, jealousy, diarrhea, acidity, ulceration, skin disorders, impotency, infertility, fainting, hiccups, tremor, weakness, emaciation, dryness, restlessness, and insomnia.

Some of the many pungent herbs and spices include Shunti (dry ginger), Sarshapa (brown mustard seed), Maricha (black pepper), Chitrak, Vidanga, and Ajwain. Katu herbs are Ayurvedic essentials for treating Kapha dosha and during times of sluggish digestion, slow metabolism, weight loss, congestion, dull mind, lethargy, and poor motivation.

Bitter—Air and Ether

Tikta is the bitter taste and manifests from Air and Ether. It has an affinity for the liver, spleen, and pancreas, and acts directly on the blood. It is cooling, drying, lightening, and catabolic (reducing). Tikta reduces Kapha and Pitta but quickly provokes Vata.

Tikta has powerful antimicrobial, antiparasitical properties that can be seen even in Western medicine through the bitter taste of antibiotics. Tikta relieves fever, inflammation, itching, skin disorders, liver conditions, and blood toxicity. It removes excessive fat, dries out mucus, improves digestion, cleanses the system, and reduces blood sugar. Bitter promotes austerity and celibacy and removes attachment and desire. Too much tikta creates a bitter, cynical mind and leads to isolation and depression. With excessive use, bitter can cause dryness, anxiety, insomnia, impotency, infertility, fainting, weakness, emaciation, and malaise.

The bitter taste reduces sweet cravings and makes food taste better. Some essential herbs are Neem, Kalmegha, Kutki, Haridra (turmeric), and Musta, which are beneficial for detoxification, digestion, liver health, parasitic infection, and most Pitta and Kapha disorders.

Astringent—Air and Earth

The astringent taste, known as *kashaya*, comes from Air and Earth. It has an affinity for the colon. Kashaya is cooling, drying, and slightly light. It balances Kapha and Pitta but increases Vata readily.

With its drying nature, kashaya helps stop bleeding and bind stools. It is an effective wound healer and decongestant. Kashaya promotes absorption of nutrients, reduces heat and inflammation, and repairs ulcers. The astringent taste encourages a clear, cohesive, and organized mind. With too much, dryness, thirst, gas, constipation, constriction, impotency, infertility, insomnia, depletion, and stiffness may arise. Mental imbalances such as inflexibility, harshness, heartache, spaciness, restlessness, fear, and anxiety can be provoked.

The astringent taste is unique to Ayurveda, as Western medicine considers it to be a reaction of the tongue. Some fundamental astringent herbs include Yashtimadhu (licorice), Haridra (turmeric), and Triphala.

The Six Tastes and Your Ayurvedic Practice

The six tastes, when used appropriately, are universally beneficial and will work to bring balance. However, when used improperly, they can lead to disorder and disease. For instance, sweet seems to bestow numerous healing properties, but it must be used in proper amounts and context. Refined sugar acts much differently from fruit or honey, and one

Discovering Ayurvedic Herbs: Ama Pachana

Another indispensable group of herbs in Ayurveda is known as Ama Pachana. *Ama* denotes toxins, and *Pachana* means "to cook" or "to burn"; hence Ama Pachana herbs detoxify the system by directly "burning" toxins.

Ama Pachana herbs are often heating, lightening, and drying to counterbalance the cool, heavy, and damp nature of Ama (toxins). Some of the most powerful include Chitrak, Guduchi, ginger, Vidanga, and Triphala. The ones you choose will depend on your personal needs. Whichever you decide, the herbs should support your dosha, digestion, imbalance, age, strength, and overall health-care needs.

Ama Pachana herbs will enhance any detox program, but they can be taken for daily health maintenance as well. While some Ama Pachana herbs are gentle enough to use long-term, others can be quite harsh and may create depletion, restlessness, sleep disturbance, and anxiety with prolonged use.

teaspoon of honey is much different from several. We all need sweet in our lives, but the question is: What are the best sources and right amounts for you?

No matter your dosha type, it is important to get all six tastes in your daily life. If you are deficient in certain tastes (especially ones for balance), herbs and spices can be a powerful way to get them in. Bitter and astringent are often lacking in the Western diet. By adding some cumin, turmeric, and cilantro to meals, you will enhance these flavors and improve the healthiness and digestibility of your food.

Herbal teas are another easy way to obtain the six tastes. Favor tastes that are specific for your health-care needs. Suppose you are a light, cold Vata type with excessive Ether and Air. Try a tea using Tulsi, Ardraka (fresh ginger), Tvak (cinnamon), and Ashwagandha. Add milk and honey and you've created a warming, grounding, sweet drink. Moving further, we will learn more about how the six tastes integrate into Ayurvedic herbal medicine in a practical way. We will also delve deeper into Ayurvedic practice, learning what dhatus and srotamsi are, how they interact, and how they form our whole selves. With that important foundational knowledge in place, we can begin exploring the herbal remedies in the later sections.

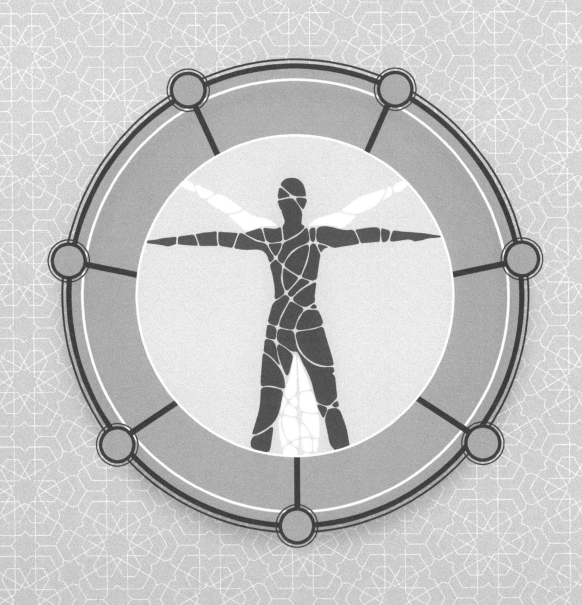

Chapter Five

☘ DHATUS AND SROTAMSI ☘

Two common terms in Ayurveda are dhatus (tissues) and srotamsi (channels). The seven dhatus are the vital tissues of the body. Together, they establish and hold together the entire system. They are life-giving, and the health of the dhatus determines the health of the individual.

A srotas is a pathway. Although there are different schools of thought, Ayurveda generally considers 14 main channels to be of most importance. Each channel has a root (mula), pathway (marga), and an opening (mukha). To maintain total health, these channels should flow freely without obstruction, misdirection, or overflow.

Becoming familiar with these structures and channels will provide you with powerful tools for your herbal practice. Each herb has an affinity for specific dhatus and srotamsi. Knowing this, you can decipher which herbs to use for the most efficient and effective treatment.

KNOW YOUR DHATUS

The seven dhatus, or vital tissues, make up our entire human system. They provide both structural and functional components. Keeping these tissues strong, healthy, and working properly is key for optimal health.

Rasa

Rasa (not to be confused with taste) is the plasma, white blood cells, and lymphatic tissue. It gives us life and brings nutrition to the entire body. Healthy Rasa is needed for optimal immunity, moist skin, energy, clarity, faith, and love. Disorders include fever, dry skin, emaciation, anemia, mental fog, edema, and lymphatic congestion.

Rakta

Rakta is our red blood cells. Rakta carries nutrients and oxygen to our tissues and waste products to the excretory organs. Healthy Rakta is needed for optimal energy, circulation, body temperature, courage, and vigor. Disorders include skin disorders, bleeding disorders, anemia, inflammation, hypertension, poor circulation, anger, and hate.

Mamsa

Mamsa is our muscle tissue. Muscles give shape to our body. They provide strength, protection, and support. Strong Mamsa is needed for body movement and gives us confidence, determination, and power. Disorders include insecurity, weakness, fatigue, flaccidity, instability, fibroids, stiffness, soreness, and fibromyalgia.

Meda

Meda is adipose (fat) tissue and consists of fats, oil, and steroids. Healthy Meda is needed for lubrication, energy, insulation, softness, and love. Too much Meda can lead to sluggishness, hypometabolism, obesity, high cholesterol, hypothyroidism, and metabolic conditions. With depleted Meda comes dryness, coldness, cracking joints, hyperthyroidism, restlessness, and rigidity.

Asthi

Asthi is our bone tissue, and it is indirectly related to nails, hair, and teeth. Asthi brings support, shape, stability, movement, and protection. Healthy Asthi requires proper nutrition and exercise. Disorders include arthritis; osteoporosis; bone spurs and scoliosis; brittle bones, nails, and hair; hair loss; and excessive cavities.

Majja

Majja consists of nervous tissue and bone marrow. Bone marrow produces stem cells, red blood cells, white blood cells, and platelets. Our nervous system governs communication, thought, feeling, perception, sensation, learning, and memory. Disorders include all neurological and mental-emotional disorders, ADHD, autism, epilepsy, tremors, anemia, poor immunity, insomnia, and restlessness.

Shukra/Artava

Shukra is the male reproductive tissue and Artava is the female equivalent. Their main job is to reproduce. They regulate sex hormones, ovulation, sexual function, and orgasm. These dhatus produce Ojas, the force behind our immunity, vitality, and libido. Disorders include low libido, impotency, infertility, premature ejaculation, and sex addiction.

KNOW YOUR SROTAMSI

Our bodies are the culmination of various pathways, or channels, known as *srotamsi*. Although they are countless in number, ancient Ayurvedic texts consider 14 to be most notable. Here, we'll address 15 in order to explore reproductive channels more inclusively. Because everything is connected in our body (and mind), keeping these channels clean, clear, and flowing freely is essential for total health.

Pranavaha Srotas

Pranavaha Srotas is the channel our life force flows through. It's often compared to the respiratory system and governs inhalation, exhalation, and communication. Its origin is in the heart (left chamber) and gastrointestinal tract, and its opening is the nose. Its pathway includes the entire respiratory system. Any respiratory condition involves Pranavaha Srotas.

Udakavaha Srotas

Udakavaha Srotas is the water-carrying channel. It provides hydration, energy, and waste removal. Its root is in the soft palate and pancreas, it flows through the gastrointestinal tract and ends in the kidneys, tongue, and sweat glands. Dehydration, electrolyte imbalance, diabetes, and edema are related to imbalanced Udaka vaha.

Annavaha Srotas

Annavaha Srotas is the food-carrying channel. It begins in the esophagus, travels through the gastrointestinal tract, and opens at the junction of the small and large intestines. Annavaha Srotas performs digestion. Imbalances include indigestion, malabsorption, nausea, and vomiting.

Rasavaha Srotas

Rasavaha Srotas includes the plasma, lymph, and white blood cells. Rasavaha Srotas bestows nutrition, immunity, and hydration. It originates in the heart (right chamber) and migrates through the lymphatic system and veins, opening where the arteries and veins meet.

Raktavaha Srotas

Raktavaha Srotas is the blood-carrying channel (circulatory system) and provides oxygen to cells. This channel includes red blood cells, the heart, liver, spleen, bone marrow, and arteries. It is rooted in the liver and spleen, flows through the arteries, and opens where the arteries and veins meet.

Mamsavaha Srotas

Mamsavaha Srotas, the muscular system, gives strength and form to our bodies. It is composed of all muscles, tendons, ligaments, fascia, and skin. Its root is in the ligaments and skin, its pathway includes the entire muscular system, and it opens at the pores of the skin.

Medavaha Srotas

Medavaha Srotas carries nutrition to the adipose, or fat tissue (Meda). This channel provides us with moisture, lubrication, insulation, softness, and love. Medavaha Srotas originates in the adrenals, kidneys, and omentum, travels through the subcutaneous fat, and ends in the sweat glands.

Asthivaha Srotas

Asthivaha Srotas, the skeletal system, consists of all 206 bones in our body and provides us with support. It begins in the adipose (fat) tissue and pelvic girdle, journeys through the skeletal system, and opens through the nails and hair.

Majjavaha Srotas

Majjavaha Srotas is the channel of the nervous system. It aligns with the nerve tissue, brain, spinal cord, and bone marrow. It offers communication and sense perception. Majjavaha Srotas is rooted in the joints. Its pathway is the entire nervous system, and it opens in the synaptic space between neurons.

Shukravaha Srotas

Shukravaha Srotas is the channel that brings life to the male reproductive tissue (Shukra). Its main goal is procreation. This channel begins in the testicles and penis, flows through the urogenital system, and opens via the urethral opening.

Artavavaha Srotas

Artavavaha Srotas carries nutrients to the female reproductive tissue (Artava). Its main purpose is reproduction. Artavavaha Srotas begins in the ovaries; travels through the fallopian tubes, uterus, cervix, and vaginal canal; and opens through the vaginal opening.

Mutravaha Srotas

Mutravaha Srotas is the urinary system. Its main functions include removing excessive water and liquid waste and providing electrolyte and blood pressure balance. This channel begins in the kidneys; flows through the ureter, urethra passage, and bladder; and opens through the urethra.

Purishavaha Srotas

Purishavaha Srotas stores and removes feces (Purisha) and relates to the colon, and it supplies nourishment via minerals. Its root is the cecum, colon, and rectum; it moves through the large intestines; and it opens through the anus.

Svedavaha Srotas

Svedavaha Srotas is the sweat-carrying channel. Its main functions are temperature control, detoxification, and moisturization. Its root is the fat tissue and hair follicles. It travels through sweat glands and opens via the pores. Disorders include scanty or excessive perspiration, body odor, burning sensations, and horripilation (goosebumps).

Manovaha Srotas

Manovaha Srotas is the mind-carrying channel. It is a vital channel for thoughts, emotions, intellect, and memory. It roots in the heart, flows through the entire body, and culminates with the sensory organs. Disorders include all emotional imbalances, mental disorders, behavioral disorders, stress, restless mind, lack of focus, and poor memory.

Discovering Ayurvedic Herbs: Agni Dipana

Agni Dipana is translated as "fire lighting." Herbs that fall into this category may be called digestive herbs, as they directly kindle the Agni, or digestive fire. Dipana herbs may solely improve digestion; however, many fall under the category of Pachana (detoxifying) as well, as these actions go hand in hand.

Dipana herbs tend to be heating, lightening, and drying, because these qualities naturally stimulate the fire element. They have an affinity for Annavaha Srotas, the food-carrying channel that relates to the gastrointestinal tract. Dipana herbs may be a necessity for just about any condition, because the root cause of all disease is an imbalanced digestive fire. Although the specific Dipana herbs you choose will vary according to your dosha and digestion type, it is often best to include at least one digestive herb in your herbal remedy.

Common Dipana herbs include ginger, Mishreya (fennel), Dhanya (coriander), Maricha (black pepper), Pippali, Jirak (cumin), and Chitrak. They can be taken in powdered form, made as an infusion, mixed with ghee (clarified butter) or honey, or added directly to food. It is often best to take Dipana herbs before a meal to prepare the Agni (digestion) for the food to come.

USING THIS INFORMATION WITH AYURVEDA

By learning the basics of these structures, you can decipher the herbal remedies that will best fit your needs. For example, if your current imbalance deals directly with a dhatu (tissue) or a srotas (channel), you can assume your disorder will involve them as well. Once you know which dhatus and srotamsi you are dealing with, you can research which herbs directly affect them. The herbs in the directory (page 47) are clearly labeled with their respective dhatus and srotamsi, making it easier to narrow your focus.

Let's put this theory into action. Suppose you are dealing with anxiety or a sleep disorder. You will look for herbs that are beneficial for Majja dhatu, Majjavaha Srotas, and Manovaha Srotas. If you have digestive issues, herbs that work on Annavaha Srotas will be best. If you have asthma, think Pranavaha Srotas; and if your goal is weight loss, Meda dhatu and Medavaha Srotas. We'll explore these varying ailments and empowering remedies in more detail in chapter 8. No matter what you seek specifically in your journey to holistic healing and wellness, we will discover together how Ayurvedic herbalism can help you.

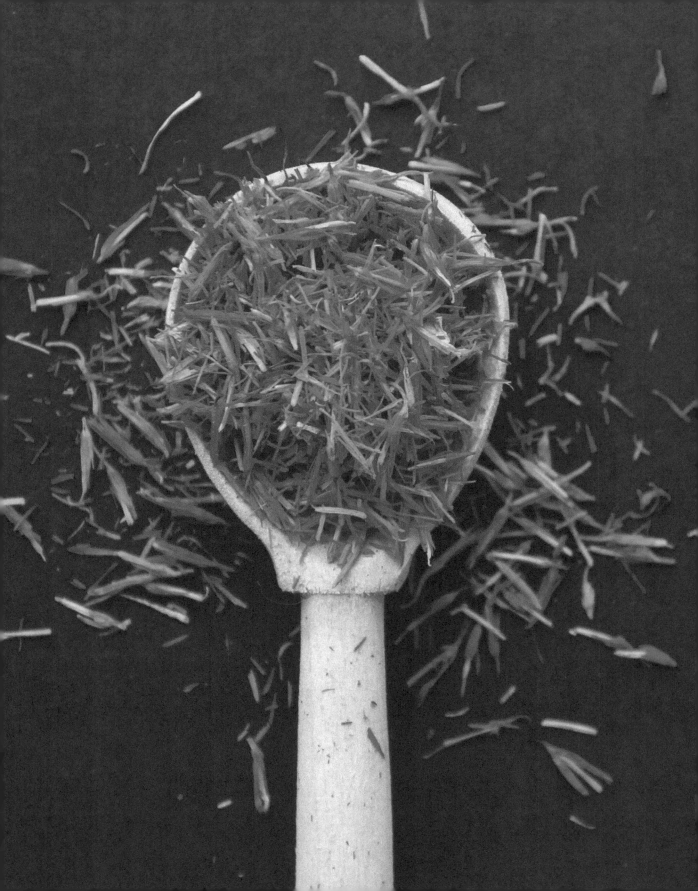

PART TWO

HERBAL DIRECTORY AND REMEDIES

Let us dive into a more practical aspect of Ayurvedic herbalism.

In part 2, we will discuss some herbal fundamentals, such as how to store your herbs, general shelf life, proper handling methods, and common preparations. Herbs are sacred in Ayurveda, so caring for them and administering them properly will ensure greater results.

Once you have an understanding of the fundamentals you can move into the Herbal Directory, a concise yet thorough look into 35 frequently used Ayurvedic herbs. With this information, you will get to know your Ayurvedic herbs, establish an intimate relationship with them, and gain confidence around using them.

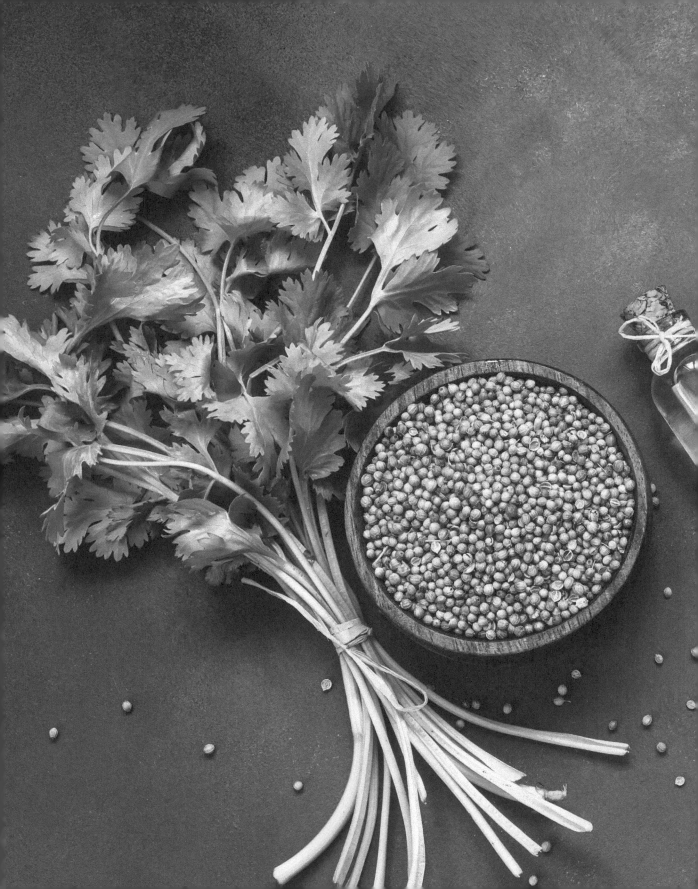

Chapter Six

KNOW YOUR HERBS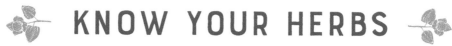

This chapter offers basic tips on getting started in your personal herbal practice, such as how to source and store your herbs. We will also discuss the various preparations used in Ayurveda, both for internal and external use. There are countless ways to administer the herbs, but you can avoid complexity and confusion by sticking to a few select herbs and simple preparation methods to begin with.

HOW TO USE HERBS

The first step is finding a reputable, sustainable, organic supplier for your herbs. Several companies offer herbs in bulk, both in powdered and whole forms. Some safe and ethical companies that I hold in high regard are listed in the Resources on page 195.

Once you start building your herbal pharmacy, store each herb in its own clean, dry glass jar. Clearly label each jar with the name of the herb and the date to avoid confusion in the future.

Keep herbs in a cool (under 70°F), dry place out of direct sunlight. With these precautions, dried herbs generally have a one-year shelf life before losing potency. Fresh herbs often need refrigeration and have a much shorter life span (three weeks at most).

Ayurveda believes plants to be holy treasures that have a mind and soul. Treat your herbs kindly! Find a dedicated area in your home for your herbs to live, ideally one that is clean, secluded, and serene. Make it your own sacred herbal temple. Play peaceful music, chant mantras, and fill this space with powerful healing energy and intention.

TOPICAL METHODS OF PREPARATION

Topical herbal preparations are invaluable for alleviating skin conditions, wounds, burns, pain, inflammation, and stiffness. The skin is the gateway to the nervous system, making these great tonics for many nervous system conditions as well. Common topical preparations include:

Medicated oils (taila)

Pastes (kalka)

Poultices (pinda sweda)

Salves

Steams (nadi sweda)

Medicated oils are easy to make, offer a wealth of health benefits, and have countless uses. These are base oils that are infused with herbs over the course of several days. They are used routinely for oil massage (Abhyanga), as well as hair, eye, nasal, and ear treatments.

Creating a medicated oil for your personal oil massage may be a nice place to begin. A self-massage with oil is performed in most Ayurvedic daily routines (dinacharya) and is useful for beautifying the skin, reducing signs of aging, and alleviating pain, inflammation, and stiffness. These massages can also be useful for calming the mind, healing the nervous system, improving sleep, and balancing the doshas.

The medicated oil you use for your self-massage should be tailored to your individual needs. Pitta types generally do best with a cooling oil such as coconut or sunflower oil, infused with Pitta-soothing herbs such as Neem, Brahmi, and Guduchi. Vata types do best with sesame oil, infused with Vata-calming herbs such as Ashwagandha and Bala. Kapha types can use a blend of sesame and sunflower oil (1:1 ratio of each oil), infused with Kapha-reducing herbs such as Punarnava, Sarshapa (brown mustard seed), and Shunti (dry ginger).

You will find various medicated oil recipes in chapters 7 and 8, including body, hair, mouth, and nose oils. The process for making medicated oils takes three days for adequate steeping time. However, the batch sizes listed for each recipe should last quite a while, even with routine use. Medicated oils will last two to three years if stored in a cool (under 70°F), dry, and dark environment.

INTERNAL METHODS OF PREPARATION

Ayurveda offers many distinct methods for taking herbs internally. Some traditional preparations include:

Cold infusions (hima)	Herbal tablets (vati)
Decoctions (kvath)	Hot infusions (phanta)
Fresh juice (swaras)	Medicated ghees (ghrita)
Herbal jellies (avaleha)	Medicated wines (arista and asava)
Herbal powders (churna)	Milk decoctions (kshirpak)

Modern preparations include tinctures, syrups, and honey infusions as well. Each preparation shifts the healing properties of the herbs, makes them more (or less) concentrated, acts on specific doshas or dhatus (tissues), or directs the remedy's potency to particular areas of the body.

Generally speaking, hot infusions (such as herbal teas) are the mildest, gentlest method for taking herbs. They are great for daily use or for those that are more sensitive to the effects of herbs (e.g., children, elderly, Vata types, pregnant people, etc.). Herbal teas can be pleasant to sip and are an enjoyable way to get your daily herbal requirements.

Herbal powders, or *churnas*, are another easy and accessible preparation. You can begin simply by combining two or three herbs that fit your current health-care needs. The herbs should be in line with your dosha, digestion and elimination type, the current season, and your level of strength. There are many methods for taking churnas, but the most foolproof way is by steeping them in warm water, stirring, and drinking (powder and all!). Although the taste is not always desirable, herbs in powdered form (rather than pill form) are more potent and better absorbed by your body.

Medicated ghees (ghritas) are unique to Ayurveda. Ghee readily extracts the properties of herbs and "drives" them deeper into tissues. Because ghee is a lipid, it can break the blood-brain barrier, making this one of the best preparations when working with brain and nervous system issues (e.g., ADHD, anxiety, depression, or sleep disorders). Medicated ghee is made by steeping herbs in water to make an herbal decoction, adding plain ghee, and steeping over a low flame until all the water has slowly evaporated out. Generally, 1 cup of herbs is used per 4 cups of ghee. The water used in the decoction will be 1 gallon per 1 cup of herbs. Depending on the size of your batch, it can take from two days to a week to complete the process.

Looking ahead to the next chapter, as well as the later sections, you will find a range of remedies that make use of these different preparations, showing just how many unique ways you can incorporate Ayurvedic herbal medicine into each aspect of your life if you so choose.

Discovering Ayurvedic Herbs: Medhya

Medhya is the group of herbs that calm, heal, and strengthen the nervous system. They stimulate the intellect, mood, focus, and memory. They are great mental tonics.

Ayurveda states that many physical disorders have a mental origin, making Medhya herbs an essential part of any herbalist's pharmacy. Some of the most well-known Medhyas include Brahmi, Shankapushpi, Ashwagandha, Shatavari, Yashtimadhu (licorice), Guduchi, Pippali, and ginger. With their ability to tone and energize, many Medhya herbs are qualified Rasayanas (rejuvenatives) as well.

Because Medhya herbs act directly on the mind and nervous system, they often do well as medicated ghee. If this is too complicated, simply taking them with ghee can be healing all on its own. A kshirpak (medicated milk decoction) can be suitable for treating sleep disorders, while steeping Medhya herbs in warm almond milk will strengthen an oversensitive nervous system. If your goal is rejuvenation, mix your Medhya herbs with ghee and honey for more effective (and tasty) results!

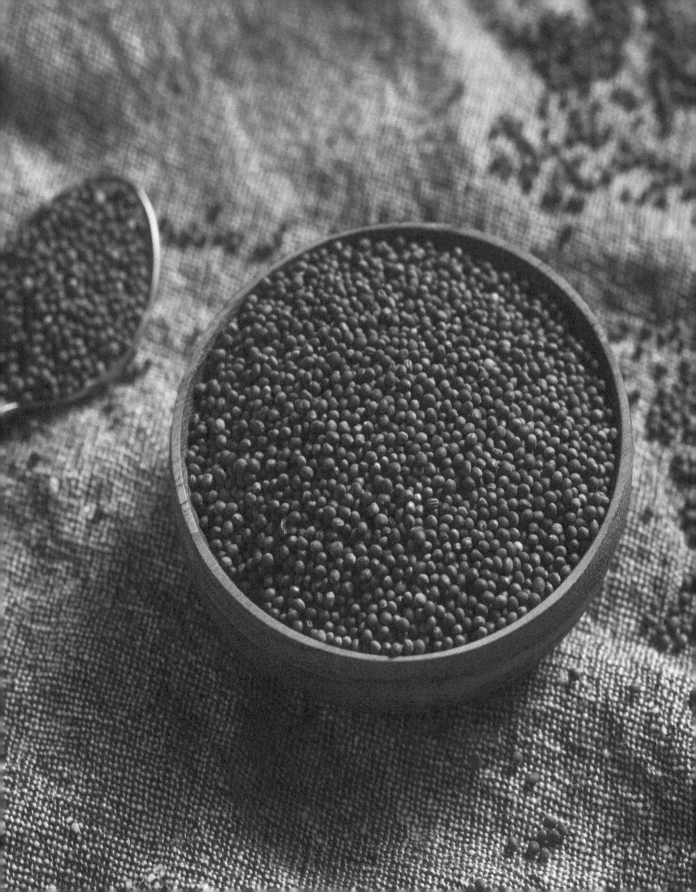

Chapter Seven

YOUR AYURVEDIC HERBAL DIRECTORY

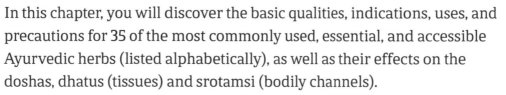

In this chapter, you will discover the basic qualities, indications, uses, and precautions for 35 of the most commonly used, essential, and accessible Ayurvedic herbs (listed alphabetically), as well as their effects on the doshas, dhatus (tissues) and srotamsi (bodily channels).

For each entry, the equal sign (=) reveals that an herb balances the listed dosha by abbreviation (V for Vata, P for Pitta, and K for Kapha), a plus sign (+) represents an increase, and a minus sign (-) means it reduces the listed dosha. With this knowledge, you can begin to use the remedies with more confidence and learn more about concocting your own herbal formulas, spice blends, teas, tinctures, oils, and more.

AJWAIN

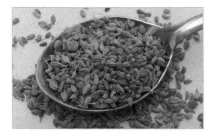

Name (Sanskrit): Ajwain
English: Carom seed
Botanical: *Trachyspermum ammi*
Part Used: Fruit (often called seed)
Dosha: VK- P+
Rasa•Virya•Vipak: Pungent, Bitter • Heating • Pungent
Prabhava: Balances five Vayus (page 6), keeps them flowing in the proper direction
Dhatu (tissue): Blood, lymph, nerve
Srotas (channel): Circulatory, digestive, nervous, respiratory, and urinary systems

Ajwain is a small seed with powerful and distinctive taste, aroma, and healing properties. Ajwain is used in recipes as a flavorful digestive spice and can help prevent indigestion. Ajwain stimulates circulation, energy, warmth, sexual potency, urination, and menstrual flow. As a nerve tonic, it relieves tension and anxiety and uplifts mood.

Indications: Ajwain relieves colic (abdominal spasm), gas, bloating, sluggish digestion, nausea, and vomiting. It is hot and penetrating, and it is useful for cough, cold, hiccups, and asthma. Ajwain is a powerful antimicrobial for parasitic, fungal, viral, and bacterial infections.

Precautions: Avoid during pregnancy, if you have a history of epilepsy, and if you are experiencing any high-Pitta conditions such as hyperacidity, peptic ulcer, and loose stools.

Cold Care Infusion

Cold, cough, fever, flu, indigestion, nausea, vomiting
Makes 6 cups

This spicy infusion is perfect when you are feeling under the weather. Ajwain targets infection, Ardraka clears congestion, Tulsi supports immunity, and Mishreya encourages digestion. For added potency, increase the water to 8 cups and steep, mostly covered, over low heat until only 6 cups remain.

6 cups water
1 (2½-inch) cube (25 grams) Ardraka (fresh ginger), finely minced
1 tablespoon Ajwain, whole
3 tablespoons cut-and-sifted Tulsi
1 tablespoon Mishreya (fennel), whole
1 to 2 tablespoons honey (optional)

1. In a large saucepan, boil the water.

2. Reduce the heat and add the Ardraka, Ajwain, Tulsi, and Mishreya. Steep on a low simmer for 20 minutes.

3. Strain and cool slightly. Stir in the honey, if using.

4. Drink 1 cup every 2 to 3 hours at first onset of cold, fever, or flu.

AMALAKI

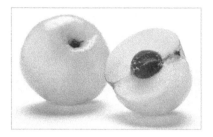

Name (Sanskrit): Amalaki
English: Indian gooseberry
Botanical: *Emblica officinalis*
Part Used: Fruit
Dosha: VPK= (V+ in excess)
Rasa•Virya•Vipak: Sour (main), Astringent, Bitter, Pungent, Sweet
  • Cooling • Sweet
Prabhava: Powerful Rasayana (rejuvenative); high in vitamin C and antioxidants
Dhatu (tissue): All seven
Srotas (channel): Circulatory, digestive, nervous, and respiratory systems; Purisha-vaha Srotas (colon)

Amalaki is one of the three herbs in the traditional herbal remedy Triphala. Amalaki is an indigenous fruit of India and contains more vitamin C than any other fruit (about 120 mg per berry). It is one of the best rejuvenating (Rasayana) herbs with strong antioxidant and immune-boosting properties. Amalaki is a mild laxative but can be taken over the long term without creating dependency. It is a natural tonic for the eyes, heart, lungs, hair, skin, brain, liver, spleen, and blood.

Indications: Amalaki is specific for Pitta digestive disorders such as hyperacidity, ulcers, inflammatory GI conditions, and hemorrhoids. It relieves constipation in large dosages (½ to 1 teaspoon) but alleviates loose stools in smaller amounts (⅛ to ¼ teaspoon). Amalaki helps reduce cholesterol, protects the heart, and is useful for anemia, arrhythmia, and tachycardia.
Precautions: Avoid during pregnancy or if you are experiencing slow heart rate (bradycardia) or loose stools (in larger dosages).

Amalaki Rasayana

Antiaging, aphrodisiac, brain tonic, eye tonic, heart tonic, lung tonic
Makes 2 cups

This rejuvenating remedy is a simplified version of a traditional formula known as Chyavanprash, *an herbal jam for supporting youth and longevity. When taken routinely, it promotes strength, energy, libido, and healthy aging.*

¼ cup Amalaki powder
2 tablespoons Ashwagandha powder
2 tablespoons Shatavari powder
1 tablespoon Brahmi powder
1 teaspoon Yashtimadhu powder (licorice)
1 teaspoon Pippali powder
1 teaspoon Ela powder (cardamom)
1 teaspoon Shunti powder (ginger)
¼ cup melted ghee (can substitute with coconut oil)
1 cup honey
2 tablespoons sesame oil

1. In a small bowl, blend the Amalaki, Ashwagandha, Shatavari, Brahmi, Yashtimadhu, Pippali, Ela, and Shunti.

2. Add the ghee, honey, and oil. Stir well until all ingredients are evenly combined and no dried herbs or clumps remain.

3. Take 1 teaspoon each morning upon awakening. Follow with a cup of warm water.

4. Store in an airtight glass jar in a dark, cool environment for up to 1 year.

ARDRAKA

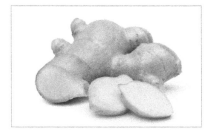

Name (Sanskrit): Ardraka (fresh); Shunti (dry)
English: Ginger
Botanical: *Zingiber officinale*
Part Used: Rhizome
Dosha: VPK= (fresh); VK- P+ (dry)
Rasa•Virya•Vipak: Pungent, Sweet • Warming (fresh); Heating (dry) • Sweet (fresh); Pungent (dry)
Prabhava: Works on all seven tissues
Dhatu (tissue): All seven
Srotas (channel): Circulatory, digestive, lymphatic, and respiratory systems

Ginger acts as a catalyst, enhancing the potency of other herbs when taken together. Fresh ginger is best for Vata and Pitta, as it is less drying and heating. Kapha does better with the hot and penetrating qualities of the dried root. Ginger can be used in its whole or powdered form, fresh or dry, and taken internally or applied externally.

Indications: Ginger is useful for gas, constipation, sluggish digestion, and slow metabolism. It stimulates digestion (Dipana) and burns toxins (Pachana). Ginger helps to alleviate inflammation, arthritis, headache, allergies, and asthma and promotes circulation, energy, and clarity. Take at first onset of cold, congestion, fever, nausea, or flu symptoms.

Precautions: Ginger is a potent blood-thinner and should be used sparingly with blood-thinning medications. Avoid if you are experiencing heat-sensitive issues such as hyperacidity, peptic ulcers, rashes, and hives.

Digestive Ginger Appetizer

Bloating, gas, slow metabolism, sluggish digestion, weight loss
Makes 1 serving

This digestive "appetizer" is taken 15 to 30 minutes before meals to stimulate Agni (digestive fire) and secretion of digestive enzymes. It is effective for symptoms of indigestion and slow metabolism, promoting absorption, and reducing gas and bloating. Take consistently for ongoing issues.

Large drop honey
1 slice Ardraka (fresh gingerroot), 1 to 2 mm thick
¼ fresh lime
Pinch pink Himalayan salt

1. Drizzle a large drop of honey onto the ginger slice.

2. Squeeze the lime over the honey.

3. Sprinkle with salt.

ARJUNA

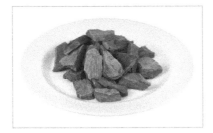

Name (Sanskrit): Arjuna
English: Arjuna tree
Botanical: *Terminalia arjuna*
Part Used: Bark (main), leaves, and fruit
Dosha: PK- V+
Rasa•Virya•Vipak: Astringent • Cooling • Pungent
Prabhava: Hridaya Rasayana (heart tonic)
Dhatu (tissue): Adipose, blood, bone, lymph, muscle (heart)
Srotas (channel): Circulatory, digestive, nervous, respiratory, and skeletal systems

Arjuna bark is named after the great warrior Arjun from the Mahabharata, indicating the strength and protection it offers. Arjuna is a well-known heart tonic that clears congestion, promotes circulation, and strengthens the heart. An effective bone mender and wound healer, it provides calcium, zinc, and magnesium. Arjuna's powerful astringency is also useful for loose stools and bleeding disorders (e.g., frequent nosebleeds and bleeding hemorrhoids). Its cooling nature soothes skin conditions such as acne, psoriasis, dermatitis, and hives, for which it can be applied externally and taken internally.

Indications: According to a 2017 article published in the *Journal of Traditional and Complementary Medicine*, Arjuna is useful for most heart conditions, including high cholesterol, high blood pressure, arrhythmia, angina, tachycardia, and heart disease. Arjuna supports healing from conditions such as asthma, anemia, obesity, tumors, osteoporosis, fractures, wounds, fever, diarrhea, bleeding hemorrhoids, heavy menstruation, UTI (urinary tract infection), bladder stones, and most skin conditions.
Precautions: Avoid during pregnancy and if you are experiencing constipation.

Arjuna Kshirpak

Broken bones, heart tonic, osteoporosis
Makes 1 cup

This milk decoction (kshirpak) is a traditional method of preparing Arjuna for its heart-healing and bone-building properties. The milk balances out its dry, astringent qualities, making it less harsh and more suitable for Vata. Kapha types will do best using almond milk instead of dairy.

> **1 cup water**
> **1 cup milk or almond milk**
> **½ teaspoon Arjuna powder**
> **1 teaspoon honey**

1. In a saucepan, bring the water and milk to a boil.

2. Stir in the Arjuna and reduce the heat to a low simmer.

3. Steep, mostly covered, until only 1 cup of liquid remains, about 30 minutes. Stir every few minutes.

4. Cool slightly. Stir in the honey.

5. Drink each night before bed to strengthen and rejuvenate the bones and heart.

6. For an easier but slightly less potent method, eliminate the water and simply heat the milk, add Arjuna, and steep for 5 minutes (stirring frequently).

ASHWAGANDHA

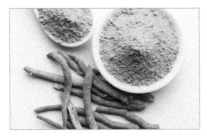

Name (Sanskrit): Ashwagandha
English: Indian winter cherry
Botanical: *Withania somnifera*
Part Used: Root
Dosha: KV- P+
Rasa•Virya•Vipak: Sweet, Astringent, Bitter • Heating • Sweet
Prabhava: Adaptogen and male reproductive tonic
Dhatu (tissue): Bone, muscle, nerve, reproductive
Srotas (channel): Muscular, nervous, reproductive, and respiratory systems

Ashwagandha is an influential Ayurvedic herb that helps reduce stress, calm the mind, tone the nervous system, regulate immunity, and strengthen the body. It boosts energy levels in the daytime and promotes sound sleep at night. Ashwagandha contains testosterone precursors, making it useful for men looking to build muscle mass, libido, and fertility; for this, it can be taken with Bala. Ashwagandha benefits women as well, and it goes well with Shatavari.

Indications: Ashwagandha is beneficial for ADHD (attention deficit hyperactivity disorder), anxiety, depression, insomnia, vertigo, Parkinson's disease, dementia, epilepsy, autism, and addiction. Ashwagandha's adaptogenic (helps body adapt to stress and promotes homeostasis) properties benefit high stress, autoimmune conditions, low immunity, and adrenal fatigue. It is useful for infertility and low libido (especially in men). Ashwagandha eases arthritis, inflammation, anemia, asthma, and muscle weakness.

Precautions: Avoid during pregnancy and if you are experiencing high testosterone conditions such as polycystic ovary syndrome (PCOS).

Ashwagandha Aphrodisiac Milk

Impotence, infertility, insomnia, low libido, premature ejaculation, weakness
Makes 1 cup

This medicated, soothing tonic destresses, calms, and soothes the nervous system. It is equally useful for enhancing libido, fertility, and sexual potency. Saffron and almonds also support reproduction and libido.

1 cup milk or almond milk
3 Keshar threads (saffron)
1 teaspoon Ashwagandha
5 almonds, soaked and peeled
½ teaspoon ghee or coconut oil
1 teaspoon honey

1. In a small saucepan, heat the milk and Keshar to just below a boil.

2. In a blender, combine the hot milk, Ashwagandha, almonds, and ghee or coconut oil. Blend on high for 30 to 60 seconds, or until mostly smooth.

3. Add the honey and stir.

4. For sleep and fertility issues, drink 30 minutes before bed. For libido, take 30 minutes before having sex (share with your partner), or as needed.

BALA

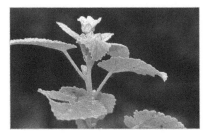

Name (Sanskrit): Bala
English: Indian country mallow
Botanical: *Sida cordifolia*
Part Used: Root (main), leaves
Dosha: VP- K+
Rasa•Virya•Vipak: Sweet • Cooling • Sweet
Prabhava: Muscle tonic
Dhatu (tissue): Muscle, nerve, reproductive
Srotas (channel): Muscular, nervous, reproductive, respiratory, and
   urinary systems

Bala is a Sanskrit word meaning "strength," and this mighty Rasayana (rejuvenative) lives up to its name. Bala builds muscle, tones nerves, enhances libido, and removes fatigue. Its heavy and moisturizing properties make it useful with high Vata. Bala strengthens the muscles, heart, lungs, and urinary system. It promotes healthy growth and development in children and healthy aging in the elderly.

Indications: Bala is supportive during weakness, fatigue, and Vata disorder. It helps with impotence, low libido, infertility, and premature ejaculation. Bala alleviates insomnia, UTI, weak bladder, dry cough, fever, asthma, and heart conditions.
Precautions: Bala contains small amounts of ephedra alkaloid and is recommended only for external use by the FDA.

Ashwagandha-Bala Oil

Arthritis, fatigue, impotence, insomnia, muscle soreness, muscle weakness, nervous system disorders

Makes 4 cups

Ashwagandha Bala Oil is a traditional formula for promoting strength and energy while reducing soreness and fatigue. This oil supports all ages and all dosha types (although it is best for Vata). You can apply this oil to localized muscles, perform a total body massage, or simply massage the scalp and feet before bed. This recipe takes three days for steeping, so plan accordingly!

> 5 cups sesame oil
> ½ cup Bala powder
> ½ cup Ashwagandha powder
> 40 drops lavender essential oil (optional)
> 20 drops Tulsi essential oil (optional)
> 20 drops orange essential oil (optional)

1. Preheat the oven to 175°F.

2. In a large oven-safe baking dish, stir the sesame oil, Bala, and Ashwagandha to combine.

3. Place the baking dish, uncovered, in the oven. Heat for 8 hours, stirring every 2 to 4 hours.

4. Let the baking dish sit for 12 hours in the oven with the heat off.

5. Remove the baking dish, stir, and repeat steps 3 and 4 twice, preheating the oven again each time. This process takes 3 days total.

6. Using a fine-mesh strainer covered with muslin cloth, strain the herbs from the oil. To get more yield, use your hands to carefully squeeze out excess oil.

7. Pour the strained oil into a bottle or jar. Stir in the lavender, Tulsi, and orange essential oils, if using.

8. Store in a dry, cool, dark area for up to 2 years.

BHRINGARAJ

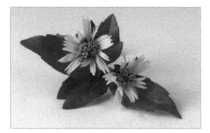

Name (Sanskrit): Bhringaraj
English: False daisy
Botanical: *Eclipta alba*
Part Used: Leaves (main), seeds
Dosha: VPK= (P+ in excess)
Rasa•Virya•Vipak: Pungent, Bitter • Heating • Pungent
Prabhava: Hair and skin tonic
Dhatu (tissue): Blood, lymph, nerve
Srotas (channel): Circulatory, digestive, lymphatic, and nervous systems

In Sanskrit, *Bhringaraj* is translated as the "king of bees," but it may be better termed "king of hair." Bhringaraj promotes healthy hair, skin, eyes, and teeth. For these, it can be used internally or applied externally. Bhriangaraj's healing properties go much deeper, however, as it protects the liver and spleen, reduces blood pressure, improves digestion (Dipana), burns toxins (Pachana), enhances memory (Medhya), purifies blood, boosts libido, and soothes inflammation.

Indications: Bhringaraj is commonly used to reduce hair loss and prevent graying. It mitigates alopecia, skin conditions, liver disorder, anemia, poor digestion, hypertension, fever, asthma, vitiligo, hernia, and headache.
Precautions: Bhringaraj should be avoided in high dosages (internal use only) with low blood pressure.

Bhringaraj Hair Oil

Alopecia, anxiety, dry hair, hair loss, headache, premature graying, skin conditions

Makes 4 cups

Bhringaraj oil can be massaged routinely onto the scalp and hair to promote hair growth, color, and luster, and applied to skin to soothe skin issues. Massaging the scalp and forehead relieves headache; massaging the feet encourages sound sleep. This oil requires three days for steeping.

2 cups coconut oil
3 cups almond oil
½ cup Bhringaraj powder
¼ cup Brahmi powder
¼ cup Amalaki powder
40 drops rosemary essential oil (optional)
40 drops lavender essential oil (optional)
20 drops Tulsi essential oil (optional)

1. Preheat the oven to 175°F.

2. In a large oven-safe baking dish, stir the coconut oil, almond oil, Bhringaraj, Brahmi, and Amalaki to combine.

3. Place the baking dish, uncovered, in the oven. Heat for 8 hours, stirring every 2 to 4 hours.

4. Let the baking dish sit for 12 hours in the oven with the heat off.

5. Remove the baking dish, stir, and repeat steps 3 and 4 twice, preheating the oven again each time. This process takes 3 days total.

6. Using a fine-mesh strainer covered with muslin cloth, strain the herbs from the oil. If needed, use your hands to squeeze out excess oil.

7. Pour the oil into a bottle or jar. Stir in the rosemary, lavender, and Tulsi essential oils, if using.

8. Store for up to 2 years.

BIBHITAKI

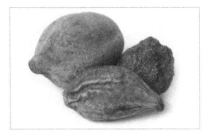

Name (Sanskrit): Bibhitaki
English: Belleric myrobalan
Botanical: *Terminalia bellirica*
Part Used: Fruit (main), seed, bark
Dosha: VPK= (V+ in excess)
Rasa•Virya•Vipak: Astringent • Heating • Sweet
Prabhava: Lung tonic
Dhatu (tissue): Adipose, blood, lymph, muscle, nerve
Srotas (channel): Circulatory, digestive, lymphatic, nervous, respiratory, and
   urinary systems

In Sanskrit, *Bibhitaki* means "removes fear from disease." Taking this herb routinely promotes longevity and healthy aging. Although tridoshic (balances all doshas), Bibhitaki is a specific Rasayana (rejuvenative) for Kapha. Being a main ingredient in Triphala, Bibhitaki works directly to cleanse the gastrointestinal tract and strengthen the Agni (digestion). It is equally as powerful as a lung, eye, skin, hair, and immune tonic.

Indications: Bibhitaki alleviates respiratory issues including asthma, cough, cold,
   congestion, sore throat, and hoarse voice. It allays many digestive complaints,
   including dyspepsia, vomiting, nausea, hemorrhoids, diarrhea, and parasitic
   infection. Bibhitaki can be used internally and externally to help relieve inflammation, hair loss, premature graying, eye conditions, skin disorders, and gout.
Precautions: Avoid with high Vata and extreme dryness conditions.

Bibhitaki Cough Syrup

Asthma, bronchitis, congestion, cough, dyspnea, laryngitis, sore throat
Makes ¾ cup syrup

Bibhitaki has a strong affinity for the respiratory system, especially when taken with "like-minded" herbs such as Pippali and Yashtimadhu (licorice). This is an essential remedy to keep in your medicine cabinet for respiratory distress.

4 tablespoons Bibhitaki powder
1 tablespoon Shunti powder (ginger)
2 teaspoons Pippali powder
2 teaspoons Lavang powder (clove)
⅛ teaspoon pink Himalayan salt
¾ cup honey
1 cup warm-hot water (per serving)

1. In a small bowl, blend the Bibhitaki, Shunti, Pippali, Lavang, and salt.

2. Add the honey and stir until no dried herbs remain.

3. Take 1 teaspoon of syrup at the first sign of respiratory illness or shortness of breath. Follow with the warm-hot water.

4. Take 3 times daily until health returns. The syrup is safe for children in ¼ to ½ teaspoon dosages.

5. Store in an airtight glass jar in a dry, cool, dark environment for up to 1 year.

BRAHMI

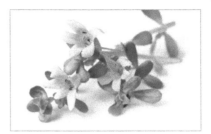

Name (Sanskrit): Brahmi
English: Bacopa
Botanical: *Bacopa monnieri*
Part Used: Leaves, stem
Dosha: VPK=
Rasa•Virya•Vipak: Bitter, Astringent • Cooling • Sweet
Prabhava: Medhya Rasayana (brain tonic)
Dhatu (tissue): All seven, especially nerves
Srotas (channel): Circulatory, digestive, lymphatic, and nervous systems and Mano-vaha Srotas (mind channel)

Brahmi works to balance emotions while stimulating intellect, focus, and memory. It is safe for all ages, supporting cognitive and behavioral development in children and healthy mental aging in older adults. Brahmi is used in many topical oils, which enable it to act directly on the nervous system via the skin. Internally, Brahmi is commonly taken as a medicated ghee, herbal tea, fresh juice, powdered herb (churna), or nasya (nasal) oil.

Indications: Brahmi is helpful in alleviating depression, anxiety, psychosis, and epilepsy. It stimulates intellect, clarity, focus, and mental development. Brahmi also soothes inflammation and relieves skin conditions, indigestion, urinary complaints (e.g., UTI, painful urination), joint pain (external), headaches (internal and external), and hair loss (internal and external).
Precautions: Avoid with bipolar disorder (may invoke a manic state).

Brahmi-Tulsi-Ardraka Infusion

Anger, anxiety, depression, foggy mind, irritability, lack of focus, memory issues
Makes 5 cups

This tasty tea is soothing to the nerves yet stimulating to the mind and intellect. Brahmi and Tulsi support healthy emotional balance and improve mental clarity and functioning. In this remedy, fresh ginger enhances these effects while stimulating Agni (digestion), as digestive imbalances play an indirect role in many mental conditions.

> 5 cups water
> 2 tablespoons cut-and-sifted Brahmi leaf
> 2 tablespoons cut-and-sifted Tulsi
> 1 (2-inch) cube (20 grams) Ardraka (fresh ginger)
> 1 to 2 tablespoons honey (optional)

1. In a large saucepan, boil the water. Add the Brahmi, Tulsi, and Ardraka.

2. Steep for 10 to 15 minutes on a low simmer.

3. Strain and let cool slightly. Stir in the honey, if using.

4. Drink 1 cup up to 3 times daily, before breakfast and between meals.

CHITRAK

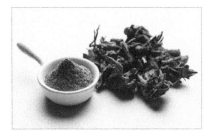

Name (Sanskrit): Chitrak
English: Ceylon leadwort
Botanical: *Plumbago zeylanica*
Part Used: Root (main), leaves
Dosha: VK- P+
Rasa•Virya•Vipak: Pungent • Heating • Pungent
Prabhava: Agni Rasayana (digestive tonic)
Dhatu (tissue): Adipose, blood, lymph, reproductive
Srotas (channel): Circulatory, digestive, lymphatic, nervous, and
   reproductive systems

Chitrak is an unbeatable herb for kindling digestion (Dipana) and burning toxins (Pachana); in fact, its alias is Agni (fire). This illustrious red root is extremely heating and renowned for boosting metabolism, facilitating nutrient absorption, and killing off parasites. Chitrak clears congestion and improves circulation throughout the body, with special focus on the lungs, liver, gastrointestinal tract, joints, and nervous system. It can be added to any formula to promote absorption but is a common ingredient in many weight-loss and digestion remedies.

Indications: Chitrak is useful when working with digestive issues such as malabsorption, dyspepsia (indigestion), loss of appetite, undue fullness, nausea, gas, diarrhea, non-bleeding hemorrhoids, weight gain, and parasites. It also works on anemia, fever, flu, inflammation, liver and spleen disorders, rheumatism, and arthritis.

Precautions: Avoid during pregnancy and when experiencing high-Pitta conditions (e.g., hyperacidity, peptic ulcer, rash, hives, etc).

Fire-It-Up Honey

Congestion, dull appetite, high cholesterol, hypothyroidism, slow metabolism, sluggish digestion, toxins, weight loss

Makes ¾ cup honey

This heating honey is a fitting remedy if your goal is stronger digestion, faster metabolism, and weight loss. Its stimulating action supports low thyroid issues, and its "scraping" quality promotes detoxification and decongestion. Take consistently for best results.

3 tablespoons Chitrak powder
2 tablespoons Shunti powder (ginger)
½ teaspoon Maricha powder (black pepper)
½ teaspoon Pippali powder
¾ cup honey
½ to 1 cup warm-hot water (per serving)

1. In a small bowl, blend the Chitrak, Shunti, Maricha, and Pippali.

2. Add the honey and stir until no dried herbs remain.

3. Take 1 teaspoon of herbal honey 15 minutes before meals and wash down with ½ cup of warm-hot water. Alternatively, this honey can be added to 1 cup of water and taken upon awakening and between meals.

4. Store in an airtight glass jar in a dry, cool, dark environment for up to 1 year.

DHANYA

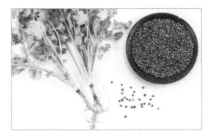

Name (Sanskrit): Dhanya (seed); Dhani (leaves)
English: Coriander (seed), cilantro (leaves)
Botanical: *Coriandrum sativum*
Part Used: Fruit (often called seed), leaves
Dosha: VPK=
Rasa•Virya•Vipak: Astringent, Sweet, Bitter, Pungent • Cooling • Sweet
Prabhava: Kindles digestion without increasing heat; removes heavy metals (leaves); potency increases with age (seed)
Dhatu (tissue): Blood, lymph, nerve
Srotas (channel): Circulatory, digestive, respiratory, and urinary systems

Dhanya and Dhani are essentials in Ayurvedic cooking and herbalism. They safely increase digestion without increasing Pitta. They also contain strong antihistamine agents and possess cooling energy. Dhani is more specific for removing heavy metals, although they both provide gentle detoxification.

Indications: Dhanya and Dhani are excellent remedies for gas, bloating, colic (abdominal spasm), hyperacidity, IBS, inflammatory GI issues, peptic ulcer, and mild detoxification. They alleviate allergies, inflammation, hemorrhoids, UTI, dysuria, water retention, hot flashes, night sweats, fever, rash, hives, dermatitis, eczema, psoriasis, cough, dyspnea, and congestion.

Dhani Juice

Allergies, detoxification, heavy metal toxicity, hot flashes, inflammation, rash, skin disorders

Makes 4 cups

Dhani Juice is a pleasant, simple drink with no juicer required. It gently flushes toxins from the system and removes heavy metals. This mild drink can be taken daily to help find relief from allergies, skin issues, hot flashes, and night sweats.

4 cups water
1 large bunch cilantro, leaves and stems, chopped
½ cup organic aloe vera juice (optional; omit during pregnancy)
Juice of 1 lime (optional)

1. Place the water and cilantro into a blender.

2. Blend on high for 1 to 3 minutes, or until the juice is completely blended.

3. If there is too much pulp, strain using a fine-mesh strainer (optional).

4. Stir in the aloe juice and lime juice, if using.

5. Drink 1 cup one or two times daily for ongoing use. During a cleanse, increase to 2 to 4 cups daily.

6. Refrigerate in an airtight glass jar for 3 to 4 days.

ELA

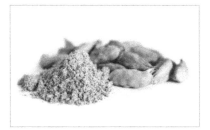

Name (Sanskrit): Ela
English: Cardamom
Botanical: *Elettaria cardamomum*
Part Used: Seeds (main), fruit
Dosha: VPK=
Rasa•Virya•Vipak: Pungent, Sweet • Cooling • Sweet
Prabhava: Kindles digestion without increasing heat
Dhatu (tissue): Blood, lymph, nerve
Srotas (channel): Circulatory, digestive, nervous, and respiratory systems

An aromatic herb, Ela is a common ingredient in spice blends, chai recipes, and herbal formulas. It is one of the few spices that kindle Agni (digestive fire) without aggravating Pitta, for which it goes well with Dhanya (coriander) and Mishreya (fennel). Being tridoshic (meaning it balances all three doshas), Ela is equally essential for soothing Vata (gas, nervousness) and clearing away Kapha (congestion, mental fog). Ela can be safely used during pregnancy to soothe morning sickness and added to coffee or tea to neutralize the negative effects of caffeine.

Indications: Ela is used to ease indigestion, gas, colic (abdominal spasm), nausea, vomiting, and morning sickness. Ela alleviates bad breath, respiratory congestion, asthma, thirst, hiccups, cough, and sore throat.

Precautions: Avoid if you are experiencing stomach or intestinal ulcers, as it may worsen symptoms.

Ela-Spiced Chai

Asthma, bloating, cold, cough, gas, morning sickness, nausea, sore throat, weak digestion

Makes 4 cups

Ela Chai is a flavorful and healing tea recipe. The aromatic spices—which can be ground using a spice grinder or mortar and pestle—stimulate digestion, clear congestion, encourage circulation, and boost mental functioning. The ample dose of Ela enhances these healing properties and eases potential caffeine spikes from the black tea. This tea is a great morning ritual to start your day with energy, clarity, and robust Agni (digestion).

> **2 cups water**
> **2 cups milk or almond milk**
> **1½ teaspoons hulled, coarsely ground Ela (cardamom)**
> **¼ teaspoon coarsely ground Maricha (black pepper)**
> **¼ teaspoon coarsely ground Lavanga (cloves)**
> **2 tablespoons black tea, green tea, or rooibos**
> **1 tablespoon cut-and-sifted Shunti (dry ginger)**
> **2 Tvak (cinnamon) sticks**
> **4 teaspoons honey (optional)**

1. In a large saucepan, bring the water and milk to a boil.

2. Reduce the heat to a simmer and stir in the Ela, Maricha, Lavanga, tea, Shunti, and Tvak sticks. Steep at a simmer for 20 minutes, stirring occasionally.

3. Strain and cool slightly. Stir in the honey, if using.

4. Refrigerate leftover chai for up to 5 days.

GUDUCHI

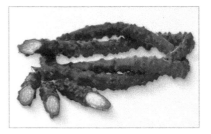

Name (Sanskrit): Guduchi
English: Heart-leaved moonseed
Botanical: *Tinospora cordifolia*
Part Used: Stem (main), bark
Dosha: VPK= (best for Pitta)
Rasa•Virya•Vipak: Bitter, Astringent • Heating • Sweet
Prabhava: Heating, but main Pitta-reducing herb; powerful detoxifier and equally
  rejuvenative
Dhatu (tissue): All seven
Srotas (channel): Circulatory, digestive, lymphatic, and nervous systems

Guduchi is one of the most commonly used herbs throughout Ayurveda's history.
Guduchi is tridoshic (meaning that it balances all three doshas) and gentle enough
to use daily and in relatively large dosages. Although heating, it is the top herb for
reducing Pitta, and despite its cleansing nature, it is one of the best Rasayanas
(rejuvenatives). Depending on your ailment, Guduchi can be taken as a powder
(churna), medicated ghee, infusion, decoction, milk decoction, or medicated oil
(external).

Indications: Guduchi alleviates specific digestive complaints including hyperacidity,
  colitis, diarrhea, celiac disease, hemorrhoids, dysbiosis (gut bacteria imbalance),
  candidiasis, and parasitic infection. It is also useful for inflammation, diabetes, fever, gout, arthritis, rheumatism, autoimmune conditions, low immunity,
  debility, mental imbalance, anemia, skin ailments, and all things liver-related
  (jaundice, hepatitis, Epstein-Barr virus, fatty liver, weak liver, etc.).
Precautions: Guduchi may lower blood sugar levels; use cautiously if you experience
  low blood sugar.

Liver Detox Kvath

Detoxification, diabetes, liver conditions, parasitic infection, skin ailments
Makes 4 cups

This remedy's powerful action is well worth its bitter taste; "bitter is better" when it comes to the liver. Take in larger amounts during liver cleanses or in smaller amounts for general liver health and maintenance. The liver plays an active role in our skin health, making this formula beneficial for skin conditions, too.

8 cups water
8 tablespoons Guduchi powder
3 tablespoons Kutki powder
2 tablespoon Haridra powder (turmeric)
1 tablespoon Pippali powder

1. In a large saucepan, boil the water.

2. Reduce the heat, stir in the Guduchi, Kutki, Haridra, and Pippali. Simmer, mostly covered, until 4 cups of liquid remain, 60 to 90 minutes. Stir occasionally.

3. Strain with a fine-mesh strainer or muslin cloth.

4. Take ½ cup (warmed) upon awakening and between meals, 3 times daily during cleanses or severe disorder. Take ¼ to ½ cup once daily for general health maintenance.

5. Store in an airtight glass jar and refrigerate for up to 7 days.

GUGGULU

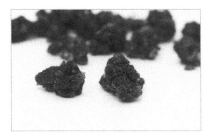

Name (Sanskrit): Guggulu
English: Indian bdellium-tree
Botanical: *Commiphora mukul*
Part Used: Gum resin
Dosha: VPK= (P+ in excess)
Rasa•Virya•Vipak: Bitter, Pungent, Sweet, Astringent • Heating • Pungent
Prabhava: Fresh Guggulu is building (anabolic); dried Guggulu is reducing
(catabolic)
Dhatu (tissue): All seven
Srotas (channel): Circulatory, digestive, lymphatic, and reproductive systems

Guggulu is the thick, aromatic sap that comes from the Indian Commiphora mukul
tree. Known for its "scraping" quality, it flushes away fat, cholesterol, and toxins.
Guggulu possesses powerful analgesic (pain-relieving) and anti-inflammatory
properties, making it useful for most arthritic conditions. It enhances digestion,
promotes elimination, and stimulates the blood, liver, thyroid, metabolism, and
immunity.

Indications: Guggulu is beneficial for weight loss, high cholesterol, thyroid conditions, edema, goiter, tumor, fibroids, cysts, low immunity, and toxicity. It
alleviates arthritis, rheumatism, and gout. It decongests and stimulates the
uterus, relieving amenorrhea (lack of menstruation), dysmenorrhea (painful
menstruation), polycystic ovary syndrome (PCOS), and endometriosis.
Precautions: Avoid during pregnancy and menorrhagia (heavy menstruation).
Use under doctor's guidance if you are on thyroid medication, statins, or heart
medications.

Slim Support Churna

Constipation, detoxification, high cholesterol, hypothyroidism, slow metabolism, sluggish digestion, weight loss

Makes 1 cup powder

Guggulu is an unbeatable asset for weight loss, and these properties are enhanced when combined with Trikatu and Triphala. Taking this churna (powdered formula) before meals supports healthy digestion, metabolism, and detoxification, but it should be taken consistently for noticeable results.

8 tablespoons Guggulu powder
4 tablespoons Triphala powder (page 136)
4 tablespoons Trikatu powder (page 93)
½ cup warm water, ginger tea, or warm honey water (per serving)

1. In a small bowl, blend the Guggulu, Triphala, and Trikatu.

2. Take ½ teaspoon 3 times daily, 30 minutes before meals. Mix in the warm water, ginger tea, or warm honey water for healthy digestion, metabolism, and elimination.

3. Store in an airtight glass jar in a dry, cool, dark environment for up to 1 year.

HARIDRA

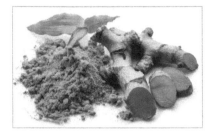

Name (Sanskrit): Haridra
English: Turmeric
Botanical: *Curcuma longa*
Part Used: Rhizome
Dosha: VPK= (P+ in excess)
Rasa•Virya•Vipak: Bitter, Pungent • Heating • Pungent
Prabhava: Blood, liver, and skin tonic
Dhatu (tissue): All seven
Srotas (channel): Circulatory, digestive, lymphatic, respiratory, and skeletal
  systems

Haridra is a renowned culinary spice and herbal medicine. It assists digestion and detoxification and boasts powerful antimicrobial, anti-inflammatory, and antioxidant properties. Haridra supports healthy cholesterol (goes well with Guggulu), blood pressure (use with Kalmegha), and blood sugar levels (try with Neem). It strengthens the blood and benefits the skin, liver, and bones.

Indications: Haridra is useful for indigestion, gas, dysbiosis (gut bacteria imbalance), candidiasis, parasitic infection, hemorrhoids, anemia, liver complaints, skin conditions, asthma, and allergies. It reduces high cholesterol, hypertension, and blood sugar and offers cancer and Alzheimer's prevention. Haridra supports women's health in amenorrhea (lack of menstruation), cramping, and uterine congestion. It is also applied topically for wounds, skin disorders, and hemorrhoids (although it stains temporarily).
Precautions: Avoid high doses during pregnancy.

Golden Milk Powder

Anemia, arthritis, dry cough, fracture, inflammation, liver conditions, sleep disturbances

Makes 1 cup powder

Golden Milk is a nighttime remedy for calming the mind, reducing stress, and encouraging sound sleep. It's a pleasant way to get in your daily turmeric dose to nourish your liver, skin, bones, blood, and brain. The supporting herbs boost digestion and reduce the heaviness of the milk, while Pippali and Maricha increase the absorption and effectiveness of turmeric.

8 tablespoons Haridra powder (turmeric)
5 tablespoons Shunti powder (ginger)
1 tablespoon Ela powder (cardamom)
1 teaspoon Maricha powder (black pepper)
1 teaspoon Pippali powder
1 cup milk or almond milk (per serving)
1 teaspoon honey (per serving, optional)

1. In a small bowl, blend the Haridra, Shunti, Ela, Maricha, and Pippali.

2. In a small saucepan, heat the milk to just below a boil.

3. Reduce the heat to a simmer and add 1 teaspoon of the herb mixture. Stirring frequently, steep for 5 minutes.

4. Pour the mixture into a mug, cool slightly, and add the honey, if using.

5. Drink 1 hour before bed each night, or as desired.

6. Store powdered herbs in an airtight glass jar in a dry, cool, dark environment for up to 1 year.

HARITAKI

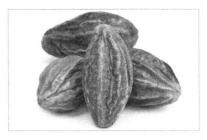

Name (Sanskrit): Haritaki
English: Chebulic myrobalan
Botanical: *Terminalia chebula*
Part Used: Fruit
Dosha: VPK= (best for Vata)
Rasa•Virya•Vipak: Astringent (main), Bitter, Sour, Pungent, Sweet
  • Heating • Sweet
Prabhava: Considered an herbal panacea with a wide spectrum of health benefits
Dhatu (tissue): All seven
Srotas (channel): Digestive, nervous, and respiratory systems and Purishavaha Srotas (colon)

Haritaki has been revered since ancient times as one of the greatest herbs for digestion, cleansing, and rejuvenation. It is called *Haritaki* because it "cures all disease" (Harayet). Considered an herbal panacea, it is one of the three herbs of Triphala. Haritaki nourishes the tissues (dhatus) to bring strength and energy while flushing out toxins, fat, and cholesterol. It is one of the best herbal laxatives, as it is gentle, effective, and can be used over the long term without side effects or dependency.

Indications: Haritaki remedies constipation (large dose), diarrhea (small dose), weak digestion, gas, hemorrhoids, and liver conditions. It is useful for parasitic infection and toxicity, as well as asthma, cough, and hiccups. It also benefits eye conditions (eyewash) and supports oral health (gargle, oil swish, or tooth powder).
Precautions: Avoid during pregnancy.

Gandharva Haritaki

Arthritis, constipation, gas, hemorrhoids, hernia, parasites, rheumatism, sciatica, toxins

Makes 1 cup oil

Gandhava Haritaki is an age-old formulation found in ancient texts such as the Bhavaprakasha (16th century CE). Castor oil (Gandharva) and Haritaki boast laxative properties that flush the colon and alleviate constipation with noticeable results. The complementary herbs improve digestion and burn toxins. This remedy balances Vata and Kapha but may increase Pitta.

> 6 tablespoons Haritaki powder
> 3 tablespoons Shunti powder (ginger)
> 1 tablespoon Vidanga powder
> 1 teaspoon Ajwain powder
> 1 teaspoon pink Himalayan salt
> 1 cup castor oil, divided
> ½ cup warm water (per serving)

1. In a small bowl, blend the Haritaki, Shunti, Vidanga, Ajwain, and salt.

2. In a cast-iron pan, heat 2 tablespoons of castor oil over medium heat.

3. Reduce the heat to medium-low and stir in the herbs and salt. Sauté for 30 seconds, stirring constantly.

4. Slowly add the remaining castor oil while stirring. Continue stirring until the oil has thickened, 5 to 10 minutes.

5. Pour the oil into an airtight glass jar.

6. Add 1 teaspoon of oil to the warm water and take before bed for up to 30 consecutive days, or as needed.

7. After 30 days, take a 1 to 3 month break (minimum) before using again.

8. Store in a dry, cool, dark environment for up to 1 year.

JIRAK

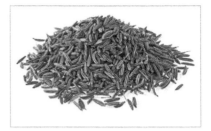

Name (Sanskrit): Jirak
English: Cumin
Botanical: *Cuminum cyminum*
Part Used: Fruit (often called seed), leaves, oil
Dosha: VPK= (P+ in excess)
Rasa•Virya•Vipak: Pungent • Heating • Pungent
Prabhava: Heating digestive, but not Pitta provoking
Dhatu (tissue): Blood, lymph
Srotas (channel): Digestive, reproductive, and respiratory systems

Jirak is a beloved spice for adding flavor, aroma, and digestibility to food. It is foremost a Dipana-Pachana (digestive-detoxifying) herb and is used in tea and herbal formulas to treat a variety of gastrointestinal complaints. Besides its ability to kindle digestion, Jirak is strengthening, scraping, and anti-inflammatory. It treats eye conditions, reduces fever, relieves pain, enhances libido, and lowers blood sugar. It is also an excellent postpartum tonic for stimulating digestion and lactation. Although tridoshic (balances all doshas), it has potential to increase Pitta, so use with care in larger dosages.

Indications: Jirak wards away indigestion, gas, bloating, nausea, colic (abdominal spasm), uterine pain, diarrhea, toxicity, parasites, congestion, and fever (chronic and intermittent). It is useful for high blood sugar, high cholesterol, and excessive fat. Jirak benefits breastfeeding and painful menstruation. Traditionally, it was also used as animal medicine.

Precautions: Avoid large dosages if you are experiencing hyperacidity and inflammatory GI issues.

Digestion Lassi

Diarrhea, dysbiosis (gut bacteria imbalance), dyspepsia, hemorrhoids, weak digestion

Makes 1 cup

A lassi is a post-meal probiotic drink common in Indian cuisine. With essential digestive spices, taking this remedy after eating supports healthy digestion and encourages optimal gut flora. If possible, use fresh, homemade yogurt for best taste and optimal health benefits.

¼ cup plain yogurt
¾ cup water
¼ teaspoon Jirak powder (cumin)
⅛ teaspoon Haridra powder (turmeric)
⅛ teaspoon Shunti powder (ginger)
Large pinch Maricha powder (black pepper)

1. In a large jar with a lid, combine the yogurt and water.

2. In a small pot or saucepan over medium heat, dry roast the Jirak, Haridra, Shunti, and Maricha for 1 to 2 minutes.

3. Add the spices to the jar and mix using a hand blender, or simply shake the closed jar until the spices are evenly blended.

4. Drink ½ cup twice daily after lunch and dinner for digestion support.

5. Refrigerate the leftovers. Drink within 1 day of making; shake well before serving.

KALMEGHA

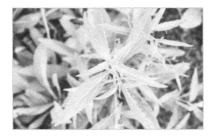

Name (Sanskrit): Kalmegha
English: King of bitters
Botanical: *Andrographis paniculata*
Part Used: Whole plant
Dosha: PK- V+
Rasa•Virya•Vipak: Bitter • Heating • Pungent
Prabhava: Extreme bitter and blood cleanser
Dhatu (tissue): Blood, lymph
Srotas (channel): Circulatory, digestive, and respiratory systems

Earning its English name as the "King of Bitters," Kalmegha is an excellent blood purifier, digestive stimulant, liver tonic, and detoxifier. It attacks unwanted microbes (bacteria, fungus, yeast, viruses, and parasites) and boosts immunity. Powerful in nature, Kalmegha should be taken in small dosages, as it is quick to provoke Vata, dryness, and depletion.

Indications: Kalmegha is useful for most liver conditions, including hepatitis, jaundice, liver enlargement, fatty liver, alcoholism, and low bile production. It allays cold, congestion, fever, flu, infection, inflammation, diarrhea, and allergies. Kalmegha mitigates parasites, Lyme disease, candidiasis, and toxicity and eases skin afflictions, hypertension, and even a sweet tooth.
Precautions: Avoid during pregnancy and if you are trying to conceive (may reduce fertility). Avoid if you are experiencing high-Vata conditions such as anxiety and insomnia.

Immunity Detox Churna

Cold, cough, fever, flu, infection, nausea, sore throat, toxins

Makes 1 cup powder

This is a powerful, antimicrobial, immune-strengthening formula that will bring relief during cold, fever, or flu. This remedy alleviates a wide range of infections and detoxifies the system for a quicker recovery. It can be taken for prevention or during illness.

6 tablespoons Guduchi powder

4 tablespoons Kalmegha powder

2 tablespoons Tulsi powder

2 tablespoons Shunti powder (ginger)

1 tablespoon Haridra powder (turmeric)

1 tablespoon Pippali powder

1 cup warm-hot water (per serving)

1. In a small bowl, blend the Guduchi, Kalmegha, Tulsi, Shunti, Haridra, and Pippali.

2. For illness prevention, add ½ teaspoon to 1 cup of warm-hot water every 3 to 6 hours at the first sign of symptoms. For alleviating illness, increase to 1 teaspoon every 3 hours, or as needed.

3. Due to the potent nature of these herbs, this formula should be used for only 30 consecutive days before taking a break (at least 4 weeks).

4. Store in an airtight glass jar in a dry, cool, dark environment for up to 1 year.

KESHAR

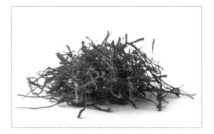

Name (Sanskrit): Keshar
English: Saffron
Botanical: *Crocus sativus*
Part Used: Stigma
Dosha: VPK= (P+ in excess)
Rasa•Virya•Vipak: Pungent, Bitter • Heating • Pungent
Prabhava: Boosts mood; reproductive tonic
Dhatu (tissue): All seven
Srotas (channel): Circulatory, digestive, nervous, and reproductive systems and Manovaha Srotas (mind channel)

Keshar carries a Sattvic (pure) quality; it balances all three doshas and promotes peace, love, and happiness. Keshar is most noted for its ability to elevate mood, calm nerves, rejuvenate tissues (Rasayana), beautify complexion, build blood, and stimulate sexual potency. As a reproductive tonic, it goes well with Ashwagandha for men and Shatavari for women. As a mood-booster, it can be taken with Brahmi.

Indications: Keshar is an excellent reproductive tonic for amenorrhea (lack of menstruation), dysmenorrhea (painful menstruation), menopause, postpartum, anemia, infertility, and low libido. It eases depression, anxiety, and a dull mind. Use internally and externally to benefit skin conditions and alleviate headache.
Precautions: Avoid during pregnancy.

Keshar-Khajoor Milk

Anemia, dry cough, infertility, low energy, low libido, postpartum, weakness
Makes 1 serving

Keshar-Khajoor Milk (saffron-date milk) is a delicious way to boost energy, mental functioning, and reproductive health. Dates are commonly used in Ayurveda as an energizing, strengthening, blood-building tonic. This drink is perfect during times of low energy, low mood, and low libido. Avoid with high toxins, congestion, or high Kapha.

7 to 10 Keshar threads (saffron)
¼ cup water
1 cup milk or almond milk
2 or 3 Khajoor (dates), pitted and chopped
¼ teaspoon Tvak powder (cinnamon)
¼ teaspoon Ela powder (cardamom)
¼ teaspoon Shunti powder (ginger)

1. Place the Keshar in the water and soak for 10 minutes.

2. Heat the milk to a low boil in a small pan; stir frequently.

3. Add the Khajoor and cook over medium-low heat for 5 minutes, or until soft; stir constantly.

4. Pour the heated milk and Khajoor into a blender along with the Keshar (and soaking water), Tvak, Ela, and Shunti. Blend until completely smooth.

5. Drink 1 cup up to 3 times weekly to rejuvenate the body, mind, and reproductive system.

KUTKI

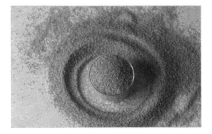

Name (Sanskrit): Kutki
English: Picrorhiza
Botanical: *Picrorhiza kurrooa*
Part Used: Root (rhizome)
Dosha: PK- V+
Rasa•Virya•Vipak: Bitter • Cooling • Pungent
Prabhava: Liver tonic
Dhatu (tissue): Adipose, blood, lymph
Srotas (channel): Circulatory, digestive, and lymphatic systems and Purishavaha
  Srotas (colon)

Kutki is renowned in Ayurveda for supporting liver health. With its unmistakable bitterness, Kutki is dry, light, cooling, antimicrobial, anti-inflammatory, digestive, laxative, and alterative (blood cleansing). Kutki acts to detoxify, strengthen, and regenerate the liver, making it useful for a wide variety of liver conditions. It is commonly used to boost immunity, destroy infection, relieve allergies, and soothe skin conditions. Its "scraping" effect flushes away fat and cholesterol, making it useful in weight loss. Due to overharvesting and unsustainable farming methods, Kutki is listed as an endangered herb—please use and source mindfully!

Indications: Kutki can be taken for hepatitis, cirrhosis, fatty liver, alcoholism, jaundice, and anemia. It is useful for sluggish digestion, slow metabolism, constipation, hemorrhoids, and parasitic infection. Kutki also acts against obesity and high cholesterol and soothes skin conditions, fever, inflammation, infection, and allergies.
Precautions: Avoid during pregnancy or if you are experiencing dryness, depletion, or high-Vata conditions.

Kutki-Aloe Liver Tonic

Alcoholism, anemia, gallbladder disorders, high cholesterol, liver disorders, skin conditions, spleen disorders, toxicity, weight loss

Makes 1 serving

This bitter tonic removes congestion, stagnation, heat, weakness, and toxicity in the liver. It acts against serious liver conditions but can be used routinely for maintaining liver health. Pippali and aloe complement the potency of Kutki and support liver health as well.

1 cup water
1 teaspoon Kutki powder
⅛ teaspoon Pippali powder
2 tablespoons organic aloe vera juice

1. Heat the water until slightly warm (not hot) and pour it into a cup.

2. Add the Kutki, Pippali, and aloe vera juice and stir.

3. Let steep for 3 to 5 minutes. Stir well and drink (do not strain).

4. Take 2 times daily between meals.

LAVANGA

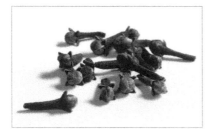

Name (Sanskrit): Lavanga
English: Clove
Botanical: *Syzygium aromaticum*
Part Used: Flowering bud
Dosha: VPK= (P+ in excess)
Rasa•Virya•Vipak: Pungent, Bitter • Cooling • Pungent
Prabhava: Extreme Pungent taste, yet cooling energy
Dhatu (tissue): Blood, lymph, reproductive
Srotas (channel): Circulatory, digestive, lymphatic, reproductive, respiratory, and urinary systems

A reputed aromatic herb, Lavanga has a vast array of uses. It clears congestion and relieves respiratory distress. It also removes sluggishness and stagnation in digestion. Lavanga increases circulation to boost energy, awaken the mind, and spark sexual energy. Its potent antimicrobial properties make it invaluable when coping with parasitic, fungal, viral, and bacterial infection. Lavanga can be taken internally as a culinary spice, herbal tea, or medicinal powder. As a pain reliever, it can be applied externally as a paste or oil.

Indications: Lavanga soothes cough, congestion, sore throat, swollen glands, asthma, hiccups, thirst, and bad breath. It remedies hyperacidity, nausea, morning sickness, sluggish digestion, malabsorption, toxicity, and parasites. Lavanga increases libido and strengthens sexual potency. It can be applied externally to relieve joint pain, muscle ache, toothache, headache, earache, and impotency.

Precautions: Avoid excessive use during pregnancy, if you are experiencing high Pitta, or while on blood-thinning medications.

Mother Nature's Cough Drop

Asthma, bad breath, congestion, cough, hiccups, indigestion, nausea, sore throat, swollen glands

Makes 1 serving

This natural cough drop brings immediate relief from persistent cough, congestion, and soreness. With its penetrating antimicrobial and anti-inflammatory properties, clove eases symptoms and eliminates microbes for a quicker, smoother road to recovery.

3 to 5 Lavanga (whole cloves)
1 cup warm water (per serving)

1. At the first sign of respiratory distress (throat tickle, scratchiness) or during sickness, suck on 3 to 5 Lavanga (whole clove buds) until they lose flavor.

2. Spit out the buds once tasteless; repeat as often as needed.

3. If this method is too intense, mix ¼ teaspoon of clove powder, ¼ teaspoon of ginger powder, and ⅛ teaspoon of black pepper powder with 1 teaspoon of honey. Slowly lick until finished. Wash down with 1 cup of warm water.

MANJISTHA

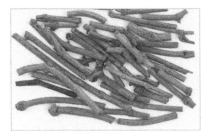

Name (Sanskrit): Manjistha
English: Indian madder
Botanical: *Rubia cordifolia*
Part Used: Root
Dosha: VPK=
Rasa•Virya•Vipak: Bitter, Astringent, Sweet • Heating • Pungent
Prabhava: Skin and blood tonic
Dhatu (tissue): Blood, lymph, reproductive
Srotas (channel): Circulatory, lymphatic, reproductive, and urinary systems

Many red herbs have a direct action on the blood, and Manjistha is no exception. Manjistha is routinely used to purify the blood, clear lymphatic congestion, and alleviate skin conditions. It kindles digestion (Dipana) and burns toxins (Pachana) to support detoxification. As an antioxidant and Rasayana (rejuvenative), Manjistha is an antiaging, complexion-enhancing skin tonic. It can be used externally to remedy skin aliments, wounds, ulcers, bone fractures, and gout. However, its red color may temporarily stain the skin.

Indications: Manjistha alleviates acne, eczema, psoriasis, leucoderma (vitiligo), rashes, and urticaria (hives). It is also a hemostatic (an agent that stops bleeding). For women, Manjistha alleviates menorrhagia (heavy menstruation), dysmenorrhea (painful menstruation), and endometriosis. It can also mitigate benign tumors, fibroids, cysts, and bladder and kidney stones, and it aids in the healing of wounds, ulcers, and broken bones.
Precautions: Avoid use during pregnancy. Use in moderation, as extreme doses cause hallucination.

Beautiful Complexion Kvath

Acne, dull complexion, eczema, psoriasis, dermatitis, hives, rash, detoxification, liver conditions

Makes 6 cups

This decoction (kvath) encourages beautiful skin from the inside out. Many skin disorders stem from high Pitta (heat) and toxins in the blood and liver. This formula eradicates these issues to pave the way for healthy skin and a lustrous complexion. You may notice your urine becomes pink while using this; don't worry! It's just Manjistha's red color coming through.

8 cups water
6 tablespoons Guduchi powder
6 tablespoons Manjistha powder
3 tablespoons Haridra powder (turmeric)
1 tablespoon Neem powder
2 cups organic aloe vera juice

1. In a large saucepan over high heat, boil the water.

2. Reduce the heat and stir in the Guduchi, Manjistha, Haridra, and Neem.

3. Simmer, mostly covered, until 4 cups of liquid remain, 1 to 2 hours depending on heat setting. Stir occasionally.

4. Strain with a fine-mesh strainer or muslin cloth.

5. Cool to around 110°F and add the aloe vera juice; stir well.

6. Take ½ cup (warmed) upon awakening and before bed.

7. Store in an airtight glass jar and refrigerate for up to 6 days.

MARICHA

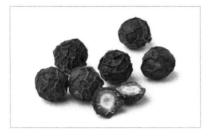

Name (Sanskrit): Maricha
English: Black pepper
Botanical: *Piper nigrum*
Part Used: Fruit
Dosha: VK- P+
Rasa•Virya•Vipak: Pungent • Heating • Pungent
Prabhava: Penetrates deep into the tissues (Tikshna)
Dhatu (tissue): Adipose, blood, lymph, nerve
Srotas (channel): Circulatory, digestive, and respiratory systems

In Hinduism, Maricha is one of the names of the sun; it translates as the "destroyer of disease." Like the sun, Maricha is sharp and heating, allowing its healing properties to delve deep into the tissues. As a stimulant, it kindles digestion, circulation, and mental functioning. Maricha burns toxins, clears congestion, and abolishes microbes. It can be used as a culinary spice, or for stronger effects, can be taken in larger amounts as an herbal infusion, milk decoction, or powder (churna).

Indications: Maricha counteracts slow metabolism, sluggish digestion, dull appetite, weight gain, toxicity, and parasitic infection. Its stimulating nature remedies poor circulation, fatigue, and a weary mind, while its affinity for the lungs alleviates cough, congestion, asthma, bronchitis, laryngitis, and sore throat. Maricha is useful as a nasal oil to mitigate infection, allergies, and headache or as a body oil to relieve aches and pain.
Precautions: Avoid high doses during pregnancy or if you are experiencing hyperacidity, inflammatory GI conditions, or high Pitta.

Trikatu Churna

Asthma, congestion, cough, high cholesterol, hypothyroidism, obesity, sluggish digestion

Makes 1 cup powder

Trikatu is a classical formula meaning three ("tri") pungents ("katu"). This combination of three spicy herbs is prescribed with Kapha imbalances such as obesity, hypothyroidism, and high cholesterol. Trikatu's heating and penetrating nature make it a powerful stimulant, expectorant, digestive, and detoxifier. It is often taken with honey to enhance its potency.

8 tablespoons Shunti powder (ginger)
4 tablespoons Maricha powder (black pepper)
4 tablespoons Pippali powder
1 teaspoon honey (per serving)
½ cup warm water (per serving)

1. In a small bowl, blend the Shunti, Maricha, and Pippali.

2. Mix ½ teaspoon of herbs with 1 teaspoon of honey.

3. Take 3 times daily 30 minutes before meals to stimulate digestion and metabolism and encourage weight loss. Follow with the warm water.

4. Alternatively, take ½ teaspoon of herbs in ½ cup of warm water.

5. For respiratory afflictions, take 1 teaspoon of herbs in 1 teaspoon of honey every 3 to 6 hours, or as needed.

6. Store the herbs in an airtight glass jar in a dry, cool, dark environment for up to 1 year.

MISHREYA

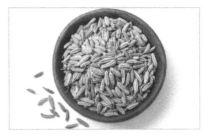

Name (Sanskrit): Mishreya
English: Fennel
Botanical: *Foeniculum vulgare*
Part Used: Fruit (often called seed), root
Dosha: VPK=
Rasa•Virya•Vipak: Sweet, Pungent, Bitter • Cooling • Sweet
Prabhava: Cooling digestive
Dhatu (tissue): Blood, lymph, nerve
Srotas (channel): Circulatory and digestive systems

Similar to its relative, Dhanya (coriander), Mishreya increases Agni (digestion) without aggravating Pitta. It is often chewed after meals to ward away gas and bloating. Fennel soothes the urinary tract and improves blood flow during menstruation. It also stimulates lactation and is an excellent friend for breastfeeding.

Indications: Mishreya benefits weak digestion, dyspepsia, gas, colic (abdominal spasm), nausea, toxicity, and hyperacidity. As a coolant, it is useful for inflammation, hot flashes, UTI, dysuria (burning urination), and menstrual cramping. Mishreya is useful during breastfeeding and postpartum, and it relaxes the nerves, relieving stress and tension.

Sweet Fennel Infusion

Digestive issues, heat, high Pitta, hot flashes, menstrual cramps, postpartum
Makes 4 cups

This sweet, cooling tea is refreshing in the heat of summer. In warm weather, it can be slightly chilled (not too cold!) but can also be taken warm or at room temperature for best results. It is quick to balance Pitta but suitable for all body types. It can be taken regularly for ongoing issues or as needed to soothe digestive upset and menstrual cramping.

6 cups water
2 tablespoons whole Mishreya
2 tablespoons whole Dhanya
1 teaspoon whole hulled Ela
5 Khajoor (dates), pitted and chopped

1. In a large saucepan, bring the water to a boil.

2. Reduce the heat to a low simmer and add the Mishreya, Dhanya, Ela, and Khajoor.

3. Steep covered, leaving the lid slightly open for evaporation. Stir occasionally until 4 cups of liquid remain, about 30 minutes.

4. Strain into a glass container.

5. Drink 1 to 2 cups daily.

6. Refrigerate the leftovers in an airtight glass jar for up to 5 days.

MUSTA

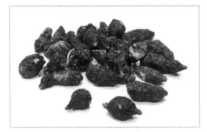

Name (Sanskrit): Musta
English: Nut grass
Botanical: *Cyperus rotundus*
Part Used: Rhizome
Dosha: PK- V+
Rasa•Virya•Vipak: Bitter, Pungent, Astringent • Cooling • Pungent
Prabhava: Liver, skin, and blood tonic
Dhatu (tissue): Blood, lymph, nerve, reproductive
Srotas (channel): Circulatory, digestive, and reproductive systems

Musta is a potent Dipana (digestive), Pachana (detoxifying) herb with special affinity for Pitta and Kapha conditions. It is a powerful blood purifier, liver tonic, anti-inflammatory, antifungal, and antiparasitic herb found in many cleansing formulas. Musta is said to harmonize the liver, spleen, and pancreas, making it effective in many digestive complaints. It tones the nerves (Medhya), and its distinctive aroma brings about a cooling, relaxing energy.

Indications: Musta eases gas, bloating, colic (abdominal spasm), hyperacidity, inflammation, toxicity, parasitic infection, and liver disorders. Women will find relief for water retention, breast tenderness, PMS (premenstrual syndrome), heavy bleeding, cramping, menopausal complaints, and hot flashes. Musta can be used internally and externally to relieve skin conditions including acne, eczema, itching, psoriasis, and dermatitis.
Precautions: Avoid during pregnancy.

Candida Care Churna

Athlete's foot, candidiasis, yeast infection, yeast overgrowth, yeast-related skin rash

Makes 1 cup powder

This herbal formula is made up of the top Ayurvedic herbs specific for eliminating Candida albicans. In fact, it is an all-around antifungal, making it effective in destroying yeast overgrowth of all varieties. When taking it for more severe yeast issues, your diet must remain strict, limiting carbs, sugars, and dairy consumption.

6 tablespoons Guduchi powder
4 tablespoons Musta powder
3 tablespoons Haridra powder (turmeric)
2 tablespoons Neem powder
½ cup warm water (per serving)

1. In a small bowl, blend the Guduchi, Musta, Haridra, and Neem.

2. Mix ½ teaspoon of herbs with the water, steep for 1 to 3 minutes and drink. Take 3 times daily before meals. For more severe infections, increase to 1 teaspoon 3 times daily.

3. Store the herbs in an airtight glass jar in a dry, cool, dark environment for up to 1 year.

NEEM

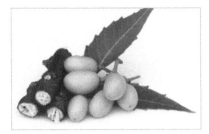

Name (Sanskrit): Neem
English: Neem tree
Botanical: *Azadirachta indica*
Part Used: Leaves (main), flower, root, bark, stem, branches
Dosha: PK- V+
Rasa•Virya•Vipak: Bitter, Astringent • Cooling • Pungent
Prabhava: Extremely bitter and reducing, yet Rasayana (rejuvenative) action
Dhatu (tissue): Adipose, blood, lymph
Srotas (channel): Circulatory, digestive, respiratory, and urinary systems

Neem is a popular herb known for its extremely bitter taste. Its cooling, anti-inflammatory properties help detoxify the liver and blood. Neem has been employed since ancient times to treat illness, infection, and parasites. It acts directly on the skin and can be applied externally as an oil or paste. Neem is a great antiseptic and holds traditional use as a toothbrush (twigs), mouth rinse (infusion), tooth powder, and oil-swish.

Indications: Neem is useful for colitis, hyperacidity, ulcers, hemorrhoids, candidiasis, and parasitic infection. It mitigates high blood sugar, diabetes, obesity, liver disorders, fever, and infection. Neem soothes skin conditions, heals wounds, and alleviates toothache, gingivitis, and mouth ulcers.

Precautions: Avoid during pregnancy and preconception (reduces fertility) or if you are experiencing high-Vata conditions such as dryness, anxiety, and insomnia.

Antifungal Foot Soak

Athlete's foot, dry feet, general foot care, itchy feet, nail infection
Makes 3 cups

Herbal foot soaks are wonderful for supporting healthy nails and feet. This antifungal blend should be used at least three days a week for severe issues, or weekly for general foot care. Foot soaks are soothing, grounding, and calm the energy after a long day.

4 tablespoons Neem powder
4 tablespoons Kalmegha powder
3 tablespoons Guduchi powder
3 tablespoons Musta powder
2 tablespoons Ajwain powder
1 cup baking soda
1 cup Epsom salt
Castor oil (optional)

1. In a small bowl, blend the Neem, Kalmegha, Guduchi, Musta, and Ajwain.

2. Add the baking soda and Epsom salt, stirring evenly until combined.

3. Add ⅓ cup of foot soak per gallon of hot water; stir until fully dissolved.

4. Soak the feet for 15 to 30 minutes. Rinse and dry the feet. If using, massage castor oil onto the feet to soothe the skin. Socks should be worn after oil application for at least 15 minutes to allow the oil to fully absorb.

5. Store in an airtight glass jar for up to 1 year.

PIPPALI

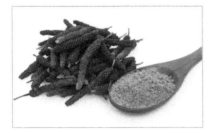

Name (Sanskrit): Pippali
English: Indian long pepper
Botanical: *Piper longum*
Part Used: Fruit (main), root
Dosha: VPK= (P+ in excess)
Rasa•Virya•Vipak: Pungent • Anushnashita (not cold, not hot) • Sweet
Prabhava: Neutral energy—not heating, not cooling; Lung Rasayana (rejuvenative)
Dhatu (tissue): Adipose, blood, lymph, nerve, reproductive
Srotas (channel): Circulatory, digestive, reproductive, and respiratory systems

Pippali dates back to around 1000 BCE, where it was first listed as a Rasayana (rejuvenative) in the Atharva Veda. It is widely used today as a lung, liver, blood, digestion, and nerve tonic. It acts on the Pranavaha Srotas (respiratory system) to remedy respiratory ailments. In the nervous system, its penetrating Medhya (nerve-calming) action pacifies Vata and calms the mind. Due to its "anushashita" (not hot, not cold) energy, Pippali sparks digestion without increasing heat. It is also called Yogavahi, as it enhances the potency of other herbs.

Indications: Pippali alleviates constipation, weak digestion, sluggish metabolism, and obesity. It is deemed useful for easing anemia, liver conditions, rheumatism, and gout. It soothes asthma, allergies, cold, cough, congestion, and sinus issues. Pippali also calms anxiety, worry, and restlessness.
Precautions: Avoid during pregnancy and preconception (may reduce fertility).

Vardaman Pippali Rasayana

Anxiety, fatigue, hyperactive nervous system, liver conditions, respiratory disorders, weakness

Makes 1 serving

Vardaman Rasayana is an ancient practice of gradually increasing the dose of an herb daily, followed by a slow reduction. This particular recipe is performed over the course of 20 days, allowing time to rebuild and regenerate tissues and bolster strength and energy. Vardaman Pippali Rasayana supports healthy aging and tones the lungs, liver, and mind. For best results, follow a nutritious, simple diet simultaneously.

1 cup milk or almond milk
½ cup water
300 whole Pippali fruits, divided
1 teaspoon honey

1. In a saucepan over high heat, boil the milk and water. Reduce the heat to a simmer.

2. Add 3 Pippali and simmer, mostly covered, until only 1 cup of liquid remains, 20 to 30 minutes. Stir every 3 to 5 minutes.

3. Strain, cool slightly, add the honey, and drink.

4. Repeat this process for 20 consecutive days. On days 2 through 10, increase the daily amount of Pippali by three each day. This equates to three on day 1, six on day 2, nine on day 3; etc. Continue this pattern until day 10, when you reach the maximum dose of 30 Pippali fruits.

5. From days 11 through 20, you will be reducing by three daily until the 20th day. For example, 27 on day 11, 24 on day 12, 21 on day 13, etc. Continue to decrease by three daily until the 20th day, when you complete this process with 3 Pippali fruits.

6. Take this remedy before eating or drinking each morning.

PUNARNAVA

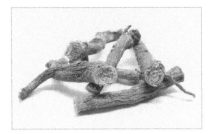

Name (Sanskrit): Punarnava
English: Spreading hogweed
Botanical: *Boerhaavia diffusa*
Part Used: Root (main), whole plant, seed
Dosha: VPK=
Rasa•Virya•Vipak: Sweet, Bitter, Astringent • Heating • Sweet
Prabhava: Main Kapha-pacifying herb
Dhatu (tissue): Adipose, blood, lymph, muscle, nerve
Srotas (channel): Circulatory, digestive, lymphatic, respiratory, and urinary systems

Punarnava is an age-old Rasayana (rejuvenative) whose name means "one that renews." Although tridoshic (balances all doshas), it especially reduces Kapha and alleviates Kapha disorders. Punarnava also acts on the liver, heart, kidneys, and urinary tract. When taken appropriately, Punarnava is deemed safe and gentle to use in (relatively) larger dosages.

Indications: Punarnava is helpful for obesity, congestion, high cholesterol, hypertension, constipation, sluggish digestion, slow metabolism, and sleepiness after eating. It also acts against diabetes, anemia, edema, water retention, UTI, asthma, allergies, and glaucoma. Punarnava relieves urinary, kidney, heart, and liver conditions, and benefits women experiencing menorrhagia (heavy menstruation), endometriosis, fibroids, cysts, and polycystic ovary syndrome (PCOS).
Precautions: Avoid during pregnancy.

Kapha-Balancing Tonic

Allergies, asthma, congestion, constipation, edema, high cholesterol, sluggish digestion, toxins, water retention, weight loss

Makes 1 cup

This tonic brings powerful Kapha-reducing herbs together to conquer Kapha imbalances of all kinds. Because the "Kapha time" of morning is 6 a.m. to 10 a.m., this drink should be taken first thing each morning during times of weight loss, allergies, congestion, or general Kapha issues.

> **2 cups water**
> **½ teaspoon Punarnava powder**
> **¼ teaspoon Shunti powder (ginger)**
> **⅛ teaspoon Maricha powder (black pepper)**
> **⅛ teaspoon Pippali powder**
> **1 teaspoon honey**

1. In a saucepan over high heat, bring the water to a boil.

2. Add the Punarnava, Shunti, Maricha, and Pippali and reduce the heat to a simmer.

3. Simmer, mostly covered, until only 1 cup of liquid remains, about 30 minutes. Stir occasionally.

4. Strain with a fine-mesh strainer. Cool slightly and stir in the honey.

5. Take first thing each morning on an empty stomach. Use consistently for best results.

SARSHAPA

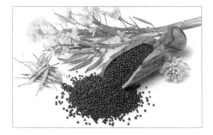

Name (Sanskrit): Sarshapa
English: Brown mustard seed
Botanical: *Brassica campestris*
Part Used: Seed, seed oil, leaves
Dosha: VK- P+
Rasa•Virya•Vipak: Pungent, Bitter • Heating • Pungent
Prabhava: Penetrates into subtle channels (Tikshna)
Dhatu (tissue): Blood, lymph, muscle
Srotas (channel): Circulatory, digestive, and respiratory systems

Sarshapa is a tiny seed with mighty potency. It is best for Kapha, as it decongests the lungs and gastrointestinal tract. As a spice, Sarshapa lightens heaviness in food and encourages digestion and detoxification. Sarshapa oil is used for Abhyanga (massage) to eliminate Kapha, increase circulation, reduce swelling, and relieve pain and stiffness. Sarshapa infusion is a useful soak for sore muscles and joints. A Sarshapa poultice can be applied to the chest to clear congestion. As a nasya (nasal) oil, it opens the sinuses and clears the mind. Sarshapa is antibacterial, antifungal, and antiparasitic to eliminate sickness and infection.

Indications: Sarshapa mitigates indigestion, slow metabolism, gas, heaviness, stagnation, toxicity, and parasites. Sarshapa also alleviates asthma, cough, and congestion. It reduces pain and inflammation to ease arthritis, stiffness, body aches, toothache, and headache.

Precautions: Avoid if you are experiencing hyperacidity, ulcer, rash, or high Pitta. Spot test mustard oil before applying to skin.

Agni Churna

Congestion, gas, indigestion, slow metabolism, sluggish digestion
Makes 1 cup

This culinary spice blend is sure to ignite Agni (digestive fire). Add to any meal to reduce heaviness and encourage digestion and assimilation. Sauté the spices in oil or ghee before adding to enliven the flavor and release their potency.

> 4 tablespoons Haridra powder (turmeric)
> 4 tablespoons Shunti powder (ginger)
> 3 tablespoons whole Jirak (cumin)
> 3 tablespoons whole Mishreya (fennel seed)
> 2 tablespoons whole Sarshapa (brown mustard)
> 1 tablespoon hulled whole Ela (cardamom)
> 2 teaspoons whole Maricha (black pepper)
> 1 to 2 tablespoons ghee or oil (per serving for sauté)

1. Combine the Haridra, Shunti, Jirak, Mishreya, Sarshapa, Ela, and Maricha in a blender or spice grinder.

2. Blend on high for 1 minute, or until the seeds have been ground into a coarse powder.

3. Place the mixture into a bowl and manually stir to ensure even blending.

4. Store in an airtight glass jar for up to 1 year.

5. To use, add ¼ to ½ teaspoon per serving in any recipe. Sauté in ghee or oil, then add spices during or after the cooking process.

SHANKAPUSHPI

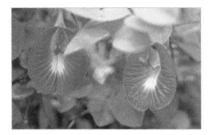

Name (Sanskrit): Shankapushpi
English: Dwarf morning glory
Botanical: *Evolvulus alsinoides*
Part Used: Whole plant
Dosha: VPK=
Rasa•Virya•Vipak: Bitter, Astringent, Pungent • Heating • Sweet
Prabhava: Medhya Rasayana (mind and nerve tonic)
Dhatu (tissue): Blood, nerve
Srotas (channel): Circulatory and nervous systems and Manovaha Srotas
(mind channel)

According to the Caraka Samhita (8th century BCE), Shankapushpi is the best of the Medhya Rasayanas (nervous system rejuvenatives). It stimulates cerebral circulation to increase intellect, memory, clarity, attention, and focus. Shankapushpi eases stress, calms the mind, and promotes sound sleep. It is an essential herb for any formula that focuses on mental health and gentle for all ages and body types. Shankapushpi also tones the liver and strengthens the heart.

Indications: Shankapushpi remedies anxiety, depression, poor memory, poor concentration, and stress. It is useful for easing epilepsy, schizophrenia, bipolar disorder, and ADHD. It relieves insomnia and strengthens a sensitive nervous system. Shankapushpi alleviates gas, constipation, liver conditions, heart disease, and hypertension.

Saraswati Churna

ADHD, anxiety, depression, lack of focus, poor memory, restless mind
Makes 1½ cups powder

Named for Saraswati, the Hindu goddess of wisdom, this classical formula is useful for easing mental conditions of all varieties. Take Saraswati with ghee to drive the healing properties deeper into the nervous system. Use ghee and honey to enhance its mental rejuvenation qualities. In the evenings, add to warm milk to promote calmness and sound sleep.

7 tablespoons Shankapushpi powder

7 tablespoons Ashwagandha powder

7 tablespoons Brahmi powder

2 tablespoons Yashtimadhu powder (licorice)

2 tablespoons Shunti powder (ginger)

2 teaspoons Jirak powder (cumin)

2 teaspoons Maricha powder (black pepper)

2 teaspoons Pippali powder

1 teaspoon Ajwain powder

½ teaspoon pink Himalayan salt

½ cup warm water, ghee, honey, or warm milk (per serving)

1. In a small bowl, blend the Shankapushpi, Ashwagandha, Brahmi, Yashtimadhu, Shunti, Jirak, Maricha, Pippali, Ajwain, and salt.

2. Mix the water, ghee, honey, or warm milk with ½ teaspoon of the herb blend. Take 3 times daily after meals.

3. Store the herbs in an airtight glass jar in a cool, dark environment for up to 1 year.

SHATAVARI

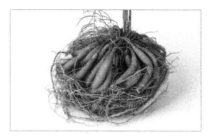

Name (Sanskrit): Shatavari
English: Wild asparagus
Botanical: *Asparagus racemosus*
Part Used: Root
Dosha: VP- K+
Rasa•Virya•Vipak: Sweet, Bitter • Cooling • Sweet
Prabhava: Female reproductive tonic
Dhatu (tissue): All seven
Srotas (channel): Circulatory, digestive, lymphatic, nervous, and (female) reproductive systems

Shatavari is a celebrated herb for female health. Its name implies "one who possesses 100 husbands," referring to the strength and beauty it bestows. Shatavari tones the uterus, regulates menstruation, balances hormones, and bolsters lactation. It supports menopause by promoting healthy estrogen. As a Rasayana (rejuvenative) and Medhya (nerve tonic), it also benefits mental imbalance, especially of a Vata or Pitta origin.

Indications: Shatavari is a female tonic and essential for amenorrhea (lack of menstruation), dysmenorrhea (painful menstruation), menorrhagia (heavy menstruation), PMS, menopause (hot flashes, bone loss, sleep disturbance, mood swings), postpartum, and lactation. It increases fertility and libido (in men, too). Shatavari relieves hyperacidity, peptic ulcer, inflammatory GI issues, and diarrhea. It also cools and calms the mind to soothe anger, irritation, and anxiety.
Precautions: Use with care during pregnancy and avoid if you are experiencing estrogen-dominant conditions such as breast cancer, fibroids, and cysts.

Shatavari Kalpa

Anger, crankiness upon hunger, excessive appetite, hot flashes, irritability, menopause, menstrual imbalance, PMS

Makes 1½ cups

Shatavari Kalpa is a traditional remedy for female health. Its cooling, soothing properties combat menstrual irregularities and menopausal symptoms. Take by the spoonful or add to warm milk for a calming yet rejuvenating treat.

3 tablespoons ghee or coconut oil
1 cup Shatavari powder
4 tablespoons date or coconut sugar (optional)
½ teaspoon Keshar (saffron)
¼ teaspoon Ela powder (cardamom)
1 cup warm water

1. In a large cast-iron pan over medium heat, heat the ghee or coconut oil.

2. Add the Shatavari and sauté, stirring constantly, until slightly brown.

3. Add the sugar (if using); stir for 1 minute.

4. Add the Keshar and Ela; stir for 1 minute.

5. Take 1 teaspoon up to 3 times daily. Follow with a cup of warm water. Take before meals to enhance the effect on the uterus.

6. Store in an airtight glass jar in a cool, dark environment for up to 1 year.

TULSI

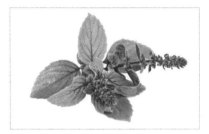

Name (Sanskrit): Tulsi
English: Holy basil
Botanical: *Ocimum sanctum*
Part Used: Leaves (main), root, seed
Dosha: VK- P+
Rasa•Virya•Vipak: Pungent, Bitter • Heating • Pungent
Prabhava: Invokes Sattva (purity), spiritual energy, and peacefulness
Dhatu (tissue): Blood, lymph, nerve
Srotas (channel): Circulatory, digestive, lymphatic, and nervous systems and Manovaha Srotas (mind channel)

Named after the goddess Tulsi (consort of Vishnu), this sacred herb bestows peace, clarity, calmness, and mental balance, purifying the mind and opening the heart. Tulsi is also an immune tonic that increases white blood cell production. It supports digestion, metabolism, detoxification, and blood sugar balance. Growing Tulsi in your home or garden is said to remove impurities, invoke purity, and bring forth auspicious energy.

Indications: Tulsi alleviates mental imbalance and reduces anger, anxiety, impurity, dullness, and fogginess. It is also useful for weak immunity, fever, cough, cold, congestion, asthma, allergies, and infection. Tulsi eases gas, bloating, colic (abdominal spasm), stagnation, and sluggishness in the gastrointestinal tract and is deemed useful for diabetes, high cholesterol, and obesity.

Immunity Tea

Allergies, asthma, cold, congestion, cough, fever, nausea, sore throat, swollen glands

Makes 6 cups

This sweet and spicy tea will ease symptoms of distress during sickness. Given its wide range of ingredients, this infusion stimulates immunity, boosts Agni (digestion), clears congestion, detoxifies, and attacks infection. Drink at the first onset of symptoms or while sick to foster a speedy recovery.

6 cups water
1 (2-inch) cube (20 grams) Ardraka (fresh ginger), finely minced and grated
4 tablespoons cut-and-sifted Tulsi
2 tablespoons cut-and-sifted Ashwagandha
1 teaspoon cut-and-sifted Yashtimadhu (licorice)
1 teaspoon whole Lavanga (clove)
3 Tvak (cinnamon) sticks
1 tablespoon honey (optional)

1. In a large saucepan, boil the water.

2. Reduce the heat and add the Ardraka, Tulsi, Ashwagandha, Yashtimadhu, Lavanga, and Tvak. Steep on a low simmer, mostly covered, for 30 minutes.

3. Strain and cool slightly. Stir in the honey, if using.

4. Drink 1 cup every 2 to 3 hours before or during sickness.

5. Refrigerate leftover tea for up to 5 days.

TVAK

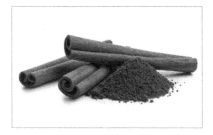

Name (Sanskrit): Tvak
English: Ceylon cinnamon
Botanical: *Cinnamomum zeylanicum*
Part Used: Bark (main), leaves, oil
Dosha: VK- P+
Rasa•Virya•Vipak: Sweet, Pungent, Bitter, Astringent • Heating • Pungent
Prabhava: Stimulates Vyana Vayu (circulation) and clears congestion
Dhatu (tissue): Blood, lymph, reproductive
Srotas (channel): Circulatory, digestive, nervous, reproductive, and
    respiratory systems

Tvak is one of the most well-known spices from the East to the West. It enlivens any dish with an aroma that awakens the appetite and the mind. Tvak alleviates digestive complaints, removes coldness and congestion, and balances cholesterol and blood sugar. Tvak eases menstrual complaints by reducing pain and cramping, regulating blood flow, and clearing obstruction. Externally, Tvak makes a great medicated oil for promoting circulation, warmth, and youthful complexion. Ancient Ayurvedic texts specifically mention Tvak as *Cinnamomum zeylanicum*, rather than its relative, *Cinnamomum cassia*, which carries different properties.

Indications: Tvak alleviates sluggish digestion, weight gain, gas, colic (abdominal spasm), diabetes, high cholesterol, candidiasis, and parasitic infection. It helps poor circulation and arthritis and relieves fever, cough, and congestion. It is also helpful for menstrual irregularities and uterine congestion.
Precautions: Avoid large dosages during pregnancy and with high Pitta.

Healthy Digestion Tea

Bloating, colic, gas, slow metabolism, weak digestion colic
Makes 6 cups

Healthy Digestion Tea can boost digestion and metabolism, prevent gas and bloating, and complement weight-loss programs. Drink in the early morning to flush the gastrointestinal tract, awaken the organs, and stimulate the mind.

6 cups water
1 (2- to 3-inch) cube (20 to 30 grams) Ardraka (fresh ginger), finely minced
4 tablespoons cut-and-sifted Tulsi
1 tablespoon whole Mishreya (fennel)
1 tablespoon whole Dhanya (coriander)
2 or 3 Tvak (cinnamon) sticks
2 tablespoons honey (optional)

1. In a large saucepan over high heat, boil the water.

2. Reduce the heat and add the Ardraka, Tulsi, Mishreya, Dhanya, and Tvak. Steep on a low simmer, mostly covered, for 20 minutes.

3. Strain and cool slightly. Stir in the honey, if using.

4. Drink 1 cup upon awakening. For severe digestive complaints, add 1 cup between meals (3 daily cups total).

5. Refrigerate leftover tea for up to 5 days.

VIDANGA

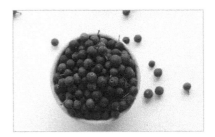

Name (Sanskrit): Vidanga
English: False black pepper
Botanical: *Embelia ribes*
Part Used: Fruit
Dosha: VK- P+
Rasa•Virya•Vipak: Pungent, Astringent • Heating • Pungent
Prabhava: Eliminates parasites and worms
Dhatu (tissue): Blood, lymph
Srotas (channel): Circulatory and digestive systems and Purishavaha Srotas (colon)

With the abundance of parasitic infections, Vidanga is a necessity for any Ayurvedic pharmacy. Vidanga has been used to combat parasites since ancient times, and its effectiveness holds strong to this day. It stimulates digestion and elimination to cleanse while killing off infection. Vidanga possesses mild antibacterial and antifungal properties; however, its true strength lies in eliminating worms and parasites.

Indications: Vidanga treats a variety of parasitic infections and is deemed safe for children in reduced dosages. It is effective against ringworm and intestinal worms. Vidanga relieves sluggish digestion, toxicity, gas, bloating, constipation, and colic.
Precautions: It may turn urine pink. Avoid during pregnancy and preconception (reduces fertility).

Para-Cleanse Tincture

Candidiasis, dysbiosis (gut bacteria imbalance), parasitic infection, toxicity
Makes 2 cups

Para-Cleanse is a harmonious formula using the top antiparasitical herbs of Ayurveda. This powerhouse remedy can be used against all types of infection, including dysentery, giardiasis, worms, and candidiasis. Take in larger dosages during a parasite cleanse or in smaller amounts for daily use. This tincture takes 28 days for proper steeping time.

> **6 tablespoons Vidanga powder**
> **5 tablespoons Neem powder**
> **4 tablespoons Musta powder**
> **1 tablespoon Lavanga powder**
> **3 cups brandy or glycerin**

1. In a small bowl, combine the Vidanga, Neem, Musta, and Lavanga. Pour the herb mixture into a 1-quart mason jar.

2. Pour in the brandy or glycerin until the liquid is an inch from the top. Cover the jar tightly and shake until the herbs are completely immersed.

3. Let the jar sit in a dark, cool environment for 28 days. Shake every 1 to 3 days.

4. Using a fine-mesh strainer covered with muslin cloth, strain the herbs from the brandy or glycerin. To get more yield, use your hands to carefully squeeze out excess liquid.

5. Fill a small glass dropper bottle for daily use.

6. Take 5 to 10 droppers 3 times daily before meals during parasitic infection.

7. Store tincture in an airtight glass jar for up to 3 years for brandy-based extract and up to 2 years for glycerin-based extract.

YASHTIMADHU

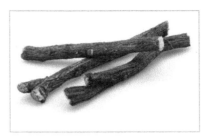

Name (Sanskrit): Yashtimadhu
English: Licorice
Botanical: *Glycyrrhiza glabra*
Part Used: Root
Dosha: VPK= (K+ in excess)
Rasa•Virya•Vipak: Sweet, Astringent • Cooling • Sweet
Prabhava: Rasayana (rejuvenative) for all tissues
Dhatu (tissue): All seven
Srotas (channel): Digestive, nervous, reproductive, and respiratory systems and Purishavaha Srotas (colon)

With its sweet, nourishing nature, Yashtimadhu is a select Rasayana (rejuvenative), Medhya (nerve tonic), Jivanya (life-promoter), and Balya (strengthener). Its soft, soothing properties rejuvenate tissues, reduce inflammation, and remove phlegm, making it useful in respiratory conditions and GI complaints. In small amounts, it reduces nausea; however, in large amounts, it induces vomiting and is a choice herb in Vamana (emesis therapy) to clear away Kapha.

Indications: Yashtimadhu eases cough, sore throat, asthma, and congestion. Yashtimadhu remedies hyperacidity, constipation, gas, ulcers, leaky gut, and inflammatory GI conditions. Yashtimadhu tones the liver, adrenals, reproductive organs (aphrodisiac), bladder, and mind.

Precautions: Avoid all use if you are experiencing kidney disease, kidney failure, heart disease, arrythmia, hypertension, or liver disease. Large dosages can lead to water retention, steroid toxicity, high blood pressure, irregular heart-beat, nausea, and vomiting. Yashtimadhu contains glycyrrhizinic acid, which may inhibit potassium absorption and increase sodium levels.

Adrenal Energy Tea

Adrenal fatigue, low energy, low immunity, mental fatigue, stress
Makes 4 cups

Healthy adrenals maintain optimal energy and hormonal balance. Chronic stress, anxiety, and overwork deplete these vital glands, leading to fatigue, lethargy, and sleep issues. This trinity of herbs rejuvenates the adrenals, calms stress and anxiety, and stimulates focus and clarity.

3 cups water
2 cups milk or almond milk
3 tablespoons cut-and-sifted Tulsi
2 tablespoons cut-and-sifted Ashwagandha
1 teaspoon cut-and-sifted Yashtimadhu (licorice)
1 tablespoon honey (optional)

1. In a large saucepan over high heat, boil the water and milk.

2. Reduce the heat. Add the Tulsi, Ashwagandha, and Yashtimadhu. Steep on a low simmer, mostly covered, for 30 minutes.

3. Strain and cool slightly. Stir in the honey, if using.

4. Drink 1 cup upon awakening and before bed.

5. Refrigerate leftover tea for up to 5 days.

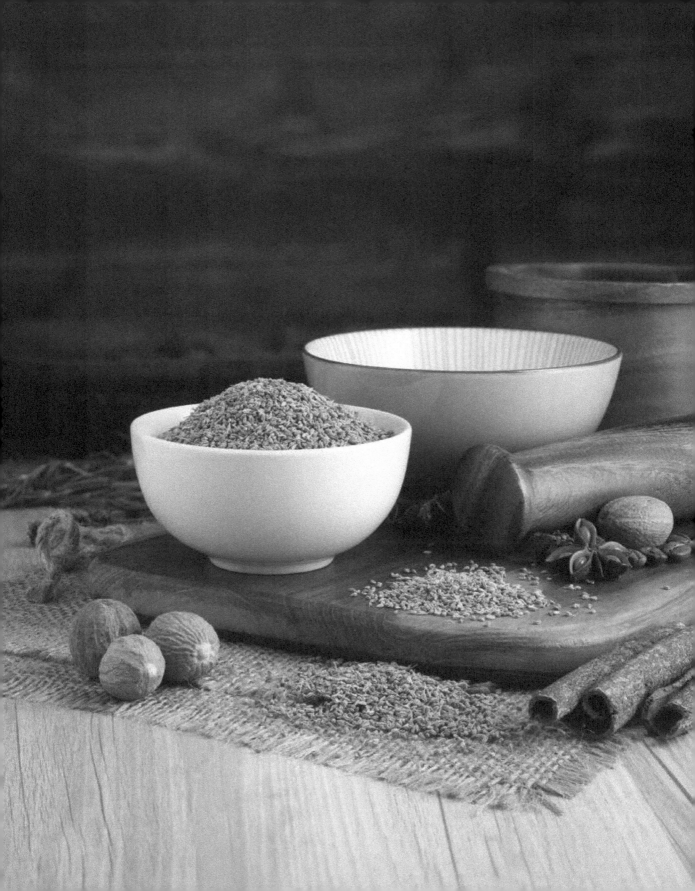

Chapter Eight

AILMENTS AND
THEIR REMEDIES

This chapter gives a brief overview of 27 common ailments through an Ayurvedic perspective. You will find some concise tips around diet and lifestyle, as these are necessary for the herbs to achieve their most optimal healing effectiveness.

This chapter includes 70 herbal recipes using the 35 herbs listed in the directory. These remedies included easy-to-make teas, churnas (powdered formulas), and tonics, as well as more involved oils, ghees, and decoctions. You'll find that each ailment has multiple remedies to give you options on your personal path toward healing.

ALLERGIES

Allergies, known as Asatmya (intolerance), are a hypersensitivity caused by weak digestion (Agni), toxicity (Ama), and depleted immunity (Ojas). Allergies display different symptoms depending on the dosha involved: Vata creates dryness and itching; Pitta, redness and inflammation; and Kapha, congestion and dullness. Dairy, sweets, and inflammatory foods will provoke symptoms and should be limited. Healthy diet, proper sleep, stress reduction, and herbal remedies will help minimize allergy flare-ups, especially if practiced consistently.

Allergy Relief Honey

Makes 1 cup honey

This pleasant-tasting remedy works wonders during allergy season. Haridra reduces inflammation, and Trikatu clears congestion and opens airways. Keep a jar handy for easy access. Drink in tea or warm water, or grab a spoonful and go! Begin this regimen 2 weeks before allergy season for optimal symptom management and prevention.

6 tablespoons Trikatu powder (page 93)
2 tablespoons Haridra powder (turmeric)
1 cup honey
1 cup warm water (per serving)

1. In a small bowl, combine the Trikatu and Haridra.

2. Add the honey and blend.

3. Store in a glass jar for up to 1 year.

4. To use, add 1 teaspoon of the honey blend to the water. Take in the morning and before bed, or as needed.

Cilantro Tincture

Makes 2½ cups

Cilantro reduces inflammation and inhibits allergic reactions. Keeping this tincture on hand is a quick, easy way to take herbs. Use consistently for chronic seasonal allergies (start 2 weeks before onset) or as needed during flare-ups. This tincture recipe takes 28 days to steep, so plan ahead before allergy season begins!

3 cups brandy or glycerin, divided
1 large bunch Dhani (cilantro), chopped
½ cup Dhanya powder (coriander)

1. In a blender, combine 2 cups of brandy or glycerin and the Dhani. Blend on high for 1 minute.

2. Pour the mixture into a 1-quart mason jar. Add the Dhanya.

3. Add the remaining 1 cup of brandy or glycerin. Cover and shake.

4. Let the jar sit for 28 days. Shake every 3 days.

5. Using a fine-mesh strainer covered with muslin cloth, strain the herbs from the brandy or glycerin. To get more yield, use your hands to carefully squeeze out any excess liquid.

6. Fill a glass dropper bottle for daily use.

7. Take 5 droppers full 3 times daily. During flare-ups, increase to 10.

8. Store tincture in a glass jar for up to 3 years for brandy-based extract and up to 2 years for glycerin-based extract.

Allergy Tea

Makes 6 cups

This tea remedy clears away allergies with its spicy nature. Ardraka, Haridra, and honey reduce inflammation, Tulsi bolsters immunity, Dhanya calms allergic reactions, and Pippali combats congestion.

6½ cups water
1 (3-inch) cube (30 grams) Ardraka (fresh ginger), finely minced
1 (1-inch) cube (10 grams) fresh Haridra (turmeric), finely minced
4 tablespoons cut-and-sifted Tulsi
1 tablespoon whole Dhanya (coriander)
2 teaspoons whole Pippali
1 to 2 tablespoons honey (optional)

1. In a large saucepan over high heat, boil the water.

2. Reduce the heat to low. Add the Ardraka, Haridra, Tulsi, Dhanya, and Pippali. Steep on a low simmer, mostly covered, for 20 minutes.

3. Strain and let cool slightly. Stir in the honey, if using.

4. Drink 1 cup upon awakening, or as needed.

5. Refrigerate leftover tea for up to 5 days.

ANGER

Anger results from high Pitta in the mind and excessive heat in the liver. It is often accompanied by irritation, criticism, and judgment. Because anger is provoked by Fire, a cooling, Pitta-balancing diet and lifestyle will often soothe the mind and release heat. Avoid hot, spicy foods, direct sunlight, extreme exercise, overwork, and stressful situations. Favor cooling foods and stress-reducing practices.

Anger Release Tea

Makes 6 cups

This soothing tea calms anger and aggression. Anger is often a reaction to stress that we tend to store deep in our bodies. When left unprocessed, it diminishes health and ruins relationships. The herbs in this blend soothe Pitta (heat) in the mind and open heart energy. Milk and dates complement the recipe with their sweet and cooling nature.

5 cups water
2 cups milk or almond milk
3 tablespoons cut-and-sifted Shatavari
2 tablespoons cut-and-sifted Tulsi
2 teaspoons cut-and-sifted Brahmi

2 teaspoons whole Mishreya (fennel)
2 teaspoons whole Dhanya (coriander)
5 or 6 Khajoor (dates), pitted and chopped

1. In a large saucepan over high heat, boil the water and milk.

2. Reduce the heat to low. Add the Shatavari, Tulsi, Brahmi, Mishreya, Dhanya, and Khajoor. Steep on a low simmer, mostly covered, for 30 minutes.

3. Strain.

4. Drink 1 cup upon awakening, or as needed.

5. Refrigerate leftover tea for up to 5 days.

Brahmi-Shatavari Ghee

Makes 2 cups

This simplified, medicated ghee recipe cools Pitta and relieves anger. Brahmi pacifies Pitta and targets the mind. Soothing Shatavari calms Pitta systemically. For severe anger and irritation, use extra ghee as a nasya (nasal oil) for instant relief and release. This ghee recipe takes three days for proper infusion.

2½ cups melted ghee or coconut oil
¼ cup Brahmi powder
¼ cup Shatavari powder

1. Preheat the oven to 175°F.

2. In an oven-safe baking dish, stir the ghee or coconut oil, Brahmi, and Shatavari to combine.

3. Place the baking dish, uncovered, in the oven. Heat for 8 hours, stirring every 2 to 4 hours.

4. Let the baking dish sit for 12 hours in the oven with the heat off.

5. Remove the baking dish, stir, and repeat steps 3 and 4 twice, preheating the oven again each time. This process takes 3 days total.

6. Using a fine-mesh strainer covered with muslin cloth, strain the herbs from the ghee or oil. To get more yield, use your hands to carefully squeeze out excess ghee or oil.

7. Pour the ghee or oil into a glass jar with a lid.

8. To use, take 1 teaspoon of ghee or oil, melted in warm milk or water, upon awakening. Take again midday or evening, if needed.

9. Store for up to 1 year, with no refrigeration needed.

ANXIETY

Anxiety is one of the most prevalent mental disorders. According to 2017 data published by Our World in Data, it affects almost 300 million people worldwide. In Ayurveda, anxiety is created by high Vata (Air and Ether) invading the mind and nervous system. For balance, we must learn to ground this "Airy" energy with calming practices such as warm, nourishing meals, hot baths, oil massage (Abhyanga), deep nasal breathing, meditation, gentle yoga, peaceful walks, and quiet time in nature.

Calm Tea

Makes 6 cups

Anxiety's pervasive energy envelops our being. This tea soothes anxious energy for calm nerves and a quiet mind. These herbs are stress-relieving nerve tonics (Medhya), and the sweet heaviness of the milk grounds energy further. This remedy is perfect for inducing tranquility at night but can be taken anytime anxiety spikes.

4 cups water
3 cups milk or almond milk
5 tablespoons cut-and-sifted Tulsi
3 tablespoons cut-and-sifted Ashwagandha
1 teaspoon whole Pippali
¼ teaspoon whole Ajwain, whole
3 Tvak (cinnamon) sticks
7 Keshar threads (saffron)
2 tablespoons honey

1. In a large saucepan over high heat, boil the water and milk.

2. Reduce the heat. Add the Tulsi, Ashwagandha, Pippali, Ajwain, Tvak, and Keshar. Steep on a low simmer, mostly covered, for 30 minutes.

3. Strain and cool slightly. Stir in the honey.

4. Drink 1 cup each evening after dinner, and as needed.

5. Refrigerate leftover tea for up to 5 days.

Calm Churna

Makes 1 cup powder

Churnas (herbal powders) are simple ways to take herbs with more potency. This formula is for balancing Vata, calming anxiety, reducing stress, and strengthening nerves. It can be taken in warm water in the daytime and in warm milk in the evenings to encourage sound sleep.

6 tablespoons Ashwagandha powder
6 tablespoons Shankapushpi powder
4 tablespoons Tulsi powder
1 teaspoon Pippali powder
½ cup warm water (per serving)
1 teaspoon ghee (per serving; optional)

1. In a small bowl, blend the Ashwagandha, Shankapushpi, Tulsi, and Pippali.

2. Add ½ teaspoon of herbs to the water 3 times daily after meals. Add 1 teaspoon of ghee, if using, for additional benefit. For severe anxiety, take 1 teaspoon of herbs per dose until balance is reestablished.

3. Store in an airtight glass jar in a dry, cool, dark environment for up to 1 year.

Tranquil Mind Milk

Makes 1 cup

This sweet, spiced milk bestows tranquility, relaxation, and peace. Milk, almonds, dates, and ghee alleviate Vata and strengthen nerves. Ashwagandha, Bhringaraj, and Shanka-pushpi are famous Medhya (mind) herbs with a powerful calming effect. Shunti, Ela, and Tvak are aromatics that will soothe your soul. Avoid with high Kapha or signs of high toxins, including heavy tongue coating, sluggish digestion, and congestion.

1 cup milk
2 or 3 Khajoor (dates), pitted and
   chopped
7 almonds, soaked and peeled
¼ teaspoon Ashwagandha powder
¼ teaspoon Bhringaraj powder

¼ teaspoon Shankapushpi powder
⅛ teaspoon Shunti powder (ginger)
⅛ teaspoon Tvak powder (cinnamon)
⅛ teaspoon Ela powder (cardamom)
1 teaspoon ghee

1. In a small saucepan over medium heat, heat the milk to a low boil, stirring frequently.

2. Add the Khajoor and cook over medium-low heat for 5 minutes or until soft, stirring constantly.

3. Put the almonds in a blender. Add the Khajoor milk.

4. Add the Ashwagandha, Bhringaraj, Shankapushpi, Shunti, Tvak, Ela, and ghee.

5. Blend on high for 1 minute, or until smooth.

6. Drink each morning, or as needed.

ARTHRITIS

Ayurveda states that the main cause of arthritis is improper diet and lifestyle habits that deplete digestion (Agni) and provoke toxicity (Ama). Once the toxins reach the bloodstream, they look for a "weakened space" in the body (in this case, the joints) and make themselves at home. The toxins soon create irritation, inflammation, pain, swelling, and degeneration. Therefore, Ayurvedic treatment for arthritis often begins with kindling Agni and burning away Ama.

Castor Oil Joint Care

Makes 1 cup

These three age-old ingredients target joints to remove toxins and reduce pain and inflammation. Castor oil is a natural detoxifier and strong laxative. If you experience loose stools, reduce the amount of oil to ½ teaspoon. This powerful recipe is not recommended to use for over 30 days consecutively. If you need long-term care, take a break every other month and try other remedies.

1 cup water
½ teaspoon Shunti powder (ginger)
½ teaspoon Guduchi powder
1 teaspoon castor oil

1. Boil the water and pour it into a mug.

2. Add the Shunti and Guduchi and stir.

3. Add the castor oil, stir well, and drink. Follow with sips of warm water.

4. Drink each night, 30 minutes before bed. Be consistent (for up to 30 days) for best results.

Arthritis Ease Churna

Makes 1 cup powder

Guggulu is a main herb in arthritis treatment. It scrapes toxins, reduces inflammation, and relieves pain. Guduchi, Haridra, and Shunti work synergistically to enhance these properties while increasing Agni (digestion). For severe symptoms, take in conjunction with the Castor Oil Joint Care (page 128) or Arthritis Ease Oil (page 130). Be consistent! This can be taken on a long-term basis, if needed.

> **6 tablespoons Guggulu powder**
> **6 tablespoons Guduchi powder**
> **4 tablespoons Haridra powder (turmeric)**
> **1 teaspoon Shunti powder (ginger)**
> **½ cup warm water (per serving)**

1. In a small bowl, blend the Guggulu, Guduchi, Haridra, and Shunti.

2. Take ½ teaspoon of herbs in water 3 times daily before meals. For severe flare-ups, take 1 teaspoon per dose for up to 2 weeks.

3. Store in an airtight glass jar in a dry, cool, dark environment for up to 1 year.

Arthritis Ease Oil

Makes 4 cups

This formula increases circulation to the joints, reduces inflammation, and eases pain. Massage this oil into the affected joints each night before bed or before a nice warm bath. It works great for sore muscles, too! This process takes three days total.

4 cups sesame oil
1 cup castor oil
6 tablespoons Guduchi powder
4 tablespoons Yashtimadhu powder (licorice)
3 tablespoons Sarshapa powder (brown mustard seed)
3 tablespoons Shunti powder (ginger)
1 teaspoon Maricha powder (black pepper)

1. Preheat the oven to 175°F.

2. In an oven-safe baking dish, stir the sesame oil, castor oil, Guduchi, Yashtimadhu, Sarshapa, Shunti, and Maricha to combine.

3. Place the baking dish, uncovered, in the oven. Heat for 8 hours, stirring every 2 to 4 hours.

4. Let the baking dish sit for 12 hours in the oven with the heat off.

5. Remove the baking dish, stir well, and repeat steps 3 and 4 twice, preheating the oven again each time. This process takes 3 days total.

6. Using a fine-mesh strainer covered with muslin cloth, strain the herbs from the oil. To get more yield, use your hands to carefully squeeze out excess oil.

7. Pour the oil into a 1-quart mason jar.

8. Store for up to 1 year.

ASTHMA

Asthma, known as Svasa in Ayurveda, is mainly a Kapha disorder, accompanied by congestion and cough. Vata may sneak in, creating dryness and constriction, while Pitta may spark inflammation. To help prevent flare-ups, avoid cold foods and drinks, sweets, dairy, refined carbs, processed foods, overeating, eating after 6 p.m., and day-sleep.

Asthma Relief Honey

Makes 1 cup honey

This sweet and spicy honey penetrates the lungs and opens the airways. Shunti and Pippali help clear congestion, and Haridra reduces inflammation. This honey can be taken regularly for ongoing issues or symptomatically during flare-ups.

> 5 tablespoons Shunti powder (ginger)
> 2 tablespoons Haridra powder (turmeric)
> 1 tablespoon Pippali powder
> 1 cup honey
> 1 cup warm water (per serving)

1. In a small bowl, combine the Shunti, Haridra, and Pippali.

2. Add the honey and stir.

3. Add 1 teaspoon to the water.

4. For prevention, take each morning and evening, with additional doses for acute flare-ups.

5. Store in an airtight glass jar for up to 1 year; no refrigeration is needed.

Breathe Deep Syrup

Makes 5 cups

Breathe Deep is a kid-friendly respiratory syrup to clear congestion, soothe inflammation, and open airways. A syrup is a decoction with a large amount of honey added to preserve and enhance potency. Enjoy this remedy "straight up," or add to warm water and sip as a tea. Be sure to never take this remedy cold.

8 cups water
6 tablespoons Punarnava powder
4 tablespoons Bibhitaki powder
2 tablespoons cut-and-sifted Yashtimadhu (licorice)
2 tablespoons cut-and-sifted Shunti (dry ginger)
1 tablespoon whole Pippali
1 tablespoon whole Lavanga (cloves)
1 to 2 cups honey

1. In a large saucepan, boil the water.

2. Reduce the heat to low. Stir in the Punarnava, Bibhitaki, Yashtimadhu, Shunti, Pippali, and Lavanga. Simmer, mostly covered, until 4 cups of liquid remain, about 1 to 2 hours. Stir occasionally.

3. Strain with a fine-mesh strainer.

4. Let syrup cool to around 110°F. Add the honey and stir.

5. Warm and take ¼ to ½ cup each morning and evening for ongoing asthmatic symptoms, or take as needed for acute flare-ups.

6. Store in an airtight glass jar and refrigerate for up to 3 months.

COMMON COLD

The common cold, or Pratishyaya, is accompanied by cough (Kasa), congestion, sore throat, and rhinitis (Pinasa; nose inflammation), showing connection with Pranavaha Srotas (respiratory system). Doshic involvement varies depending on symptoms. With white mucus, wet cough, and dull appetite, think Kapha. With fever, burning throat, and yellow mucus, assume Pitta. If you have dry cough, chest constriction, dehydration, and weakness, Vata prevails. Remember, getting sick is our body telling us to slow down.

Ginger Tea Tonic

Makes 6 cups

This potent brew will ease your symptoms and send you on a quick road to recovery. A strong dose of Ardraka and Maricha cuts through congestion, Haridra targets unwanted microbes, and lemon supplies vitamin C.

6½ cups water
1 teaspoon freshly ground Maricha (black pepper)
1 (3-inch) cube (30 grams) Ardraka (fresh ginger), finely minced
1 (1-inch) cube (10 grams) fresh Haridra (turmeric), finely minced,
    or ½ teaspoon powder
Juice of 1 lemon
2 tablespoons honey (optional)

1. In a large saucepan over high heat, boil the water.

2. Reduce the heat to low and add the Maricha, Ardraka, and Haridra. Steep on a low simmer for 20 to 30 minutes, mostly covered.

3. Strain and cool slightly. Stir in the lemon and honey, if using.

4. Drink 1 cup every 2 to 3 hours at the first onset of cold, cough, fever, or flu.

5. Refrigerate leftover tea for up to 5 days.

Fresh Ginger Flu Shot

Makes 1 serving

Fresh Ardraka juice penetrates congestion, eliminates microbes, stimulates digestion, induces sweating, and gets the blood pumping. Taking this in shot form brings tangible results and quick relief. The tonic option is equally as powerful, but less intense.

> 1 to 2 tablespoons Ardraka juice (fresh ginger)
> ¾ teaspoon freshly squeezed lemon juice
> ¾ teaspoon apple cider vinegar
> ⅛ teaspoon freshly ground Maricha (black pepper)
> 1 teaspoon honey
> 1 cup warm water

1. In a mug, combine the Ardraka juice, lemon juice, apple cider vinegar, Maricha, and honey. Stir well until the honey dissolves.

2. Option 1: Take as a shot, then follow with a cup of warm water.

3. Option 2: Add the warm water to the mug; enjoy as a tonic.

4. During illness (or for prevention), take every 2 to 6 hours as needed.

Soothing Sore Throat Gargle

Makes 1 cup

Sore throats can make it painful to talk, swallow, and sleep. This Ayurvedic gargle remedies a sore throat directly by locally destroying infection, reducing inflammation, soothing irritation, clearing congestion, and easing pain. Begin use at the first tickle, and increase repetitions if soreness worsens. Because sickness tends to flare up while sleeping, use before bed to encourage restful sleep.

1 cup warm water
1 teaspoon Haridra powder (turmeric)
½ teaspoon Yashtimadhu powder (licorice)
½ teaspoon Haritaki powder
1 teaspoon pink Himalayan salt

1. Combine the warm water, Haridra, Yashtimadhu, Haritaki, and salt.

2. Stir well until fully dissolved.

3. Take a moderate sip and gargle for 10 to 20 seconds. Spit out.

4. For severe soreness, repeat 1 to 4 times.

5. Use within 24 hours, then make a fresh batch. Cut the recipe in half if needed.

CONSTIPATION

Everyone should have one to two easeful, fulfilling bowel movements daily. Constipation is called Krura Koshta, meaning "hard stool," and reveals high Vata in the colon. It is provoked by dehydration; raw, cold, or hard-to-digest foods; poor diet; stress; anxiety; insomnia; irregular routine; and travel. For relief, keep your diet warm, well-cooked, and simple and your daily routine stable, with regular eating and sleeping times, stress-reducing practices, and plenty of warm water.

Triphala Churna

Makes ¾ cup powder

Triphala ("three fruits") is one of the most widely used traditional formulas in Ayurveda. It is tridoshic (balances all doshas), as Haritaki balances Vata, Amalaki soothes Pitta, and Bibhitaki removes Kapha. Together, this trio cleanses the gastrointestinal tract, tones the liver, and stimulates the bowels. Triphala is also an excellent long-term herbal laxative, as it doesn't create dependency or side effects.

4 tablespoons Haritaki powder
4 tablespoons Amalaki powder
4 tablespoons Bibhitaki powder
½ cup warm water (per serving)
1 teaspoon honey (optional)

1. In a small bowl, blend the Haritaki, Amalaki, and Bibhitaki.

2. Steep ½ to 1 teaspoon of herb mixture in the water. Take nightly before bed. If the taste is too strong, add the honey as needed.

3. For severe constipation, repeat in the morning. Wait at least 30 minutes to eat.

4. Store in an airtight glass jar in a dry, cool, dark environment for up to 1 year.

Haritaki Honey

Makes 1 cup honey

This honey blend is a quick, easy, and tasty way to enhance digestion and get the bowels flowing. Haritaki is a main herb for Vata conditons, including constipation. Amalaki is a mild laxative and lends a helping hand. Yashtimadhu lubricates the colon, and Shunti provides a little stimulation. This safe, gentle, and nondependent formula is suitable for all ages and long-term use.

5 tablespoons Haritaki powder
3 tablespoons Amalaki powder
1 tablespoon Yashtimadhu powder (licorice)
1 tablespoon Shunti powder (ginger)
1 cup honey
1 cup warm water (per serving)

1. In a small bowl, blend the Haritaki, Amalaki, Yashtimadhu, and Shunti.

2. Add the honey and blend evenly.

3. Take 1 teaspoon each morning and before bed. Follow with the water. Temporarily take a double dosage during severe flare-ups.

4. Store in an airtight glass jar for up to 1 year; no refrigeration is needed.

Yashtimadhu-Khajoor Milk

Makes ½ cup

This soothing nighttime drink is a mild constipation remedy. Warm milk and ghee get things moving. The herbs lubricate and stimulate the colon. Fiber-rich Khajoor encourages elimination. This milk is gentle enough for pregnancy and postpartum, but omit the Yashtimadhu and Pippali and reduce the Shunti to ⅛ teaspoon. Avoid with high Kapha or signs of high toxins, including heavy tongue coating, sluggish digestion, and congestion.

1 cup milk or almond milk
2 Khajoor (dates), pitted and chopped
¾ teaspoon Yashtimadhu powder (licorice)
½ teaspoon Shunti powder (ginger)
⅛ teaspoon Pippali powder
1 teaspoon ghee

1. In a small saucepan over high heat, heat the milk to a low boil. Stir frequently.

2. Add the Khajoor and cook over medium-low heat for 5 minutes or until soft, stirring constantly.

3. Pour the mixture into a blender; add the Yashtimadhu, Shunti, Pippali, and ghee. Blend until smooth.

4. Drink before bed for healthy morning bowels.

DEPRESSION

Depression generally denotes high Kapha in the mind and is accompanied by heaviness, lethargy, and sluggish digestion. A heavy diet, overeating, late eating, excessive sleep, and sedentary lifestyle provoke Kapha and fosters depression. Keep your diet light and healthy, limiting sweets, dairy, carbs, and processed foods. Wake up before 6 a.m. (which begins the "Kapha time") and start your day with hot water. Avoid napping and eating after 6 p.m. and get plenty of exercise.

Brahmi Bliss Tea

Makes 6 cups

Depression creates heaviness in the mind. This herbal blend will lighten your spirit. Tulsi opens the heart, Brahmi awakens the mind, Ashwagandha reduces stress, rose uplifts energy, and Keshar boosts mood. With a sweet touch of honey, this tea will make you eager to find your bliss.

6 cups water
3 tablespoons cut-and-sifted Tulsi
2 tablespoons cut-and-sifted Brahmi
1 tablespoon cut-and-sifted Ashwagandha
1 tablespoon whole rose petals (optional)
10 Keshar threads (saffron)
1 to 2 tablespoons honey

1. In a large saucepan, boil the water.

2. Reduce the heat to low; add the Tulsi, Brahmi, Ashwagandha, rose (if using), and Keshar. Steep on a low simmer, mostly covered, for 15 minutes.

3. Strain and cool slightly. Stir in the honey.

4. Drink 1 cup daily around 6 a.m. Repeat as needed throughout the day.

5. Refrigerate leftover tea for up to 5 days.

Keshar Ka Paani

Makes 1 cup

Keshar Ka Paani, or saffron water, is an age-old Indian remedy. Keshar is a brain tonic that enlivens mood. As a natural energizer, it penetrates deep to revitalize body and mind. Use consistently for best results, especially with chronic depression. You may be pleasantly surprised to find your hair and skin become more lustrous, too!

1 cup water
7 to 10 Keshar threads (saffron)

1. In a large saucepan, boil the water. Remove from heat.

2. Add the Keshar. Steep for 10 to 20 minutes; do not strain.

3. Drink 1 cup each morning around 6 a.m. For severe depression, repeat as needed throughout the day.

DIARRHEA

Diarrhea (Atisar) results from high Pitta, heat, and inflammation in the colon. Symptoms include watery stools, undigested food, frequent movements, and urgency. Whether caused by colitis, IBS, an acute illness, or chronic loose stools (Mrdu Kostha), diarrhea can lead to dehydration and malabsorption. Adopt a Pitta-soothing diet and avoid hot, spicy, oily, raw, and fermented foods. Common stool binders include cooked apple, basmati rice, ground flaxseed, ripe banana, and psyllium husk.

Dahi Shali

Makes 1 serving

Dahi Shali, or "curd rice," is a traditional remedy for easing loose or watery stools. Yogurt encourages healthy gut flora, provides nourishment, and soothes the mucosal membrane. Rice binds and is easy to digest while the Agni (gastric fire) is weak. The herbs kindle digestion and solidify the stool. Cool the rice before adding the yogurt, as the vital probiotics can die off with excessive heat exposure.

¼ **cup Dahi (curd or plain yogurt; homemade, if possible)**
1 **cup basmati rice, cooked**
½ **teaspoon ghee, melted**
½ **teaspoon Guduchi powder**
¼ **teaspoon Yashtimadhu powder (licorice)**
⅛ **teaspoon Ela powder (cardamom)**

1. Add the yogurt to the basmati rice. The rice should be lukewarm but not hot.

2. Stir until evenly combined.

3. Stir in the ghee, Guduchi, Yashtimadhu, and Ela.

4. Eat as needed during acute diarrhea. For chronic loose stools, take daily until remedied.

Flaxseed Binder

Makes 1 serving

Atasi (flaxseed) eases both diarrhea and constipation. In larger amounts, Atasi absorbs excessive liquid in the colon and binds stool. Shatavari cools heat and soothes inflammation. Shunti and Ela spark digestion. Dahi (yogurt) remedies the gut flora with a vital dose of probiotics.

¼ cup Dahi (curd or plain yogurt; homemade, if possible)
1 to 2 tablespoons freshly ground Atasi (flaxseed)
½ teaspoon Shatavari powder
¼ teaspoon Shunti powder (ginger)
⅛ teaspoon Ela powder (cardamom)
1 teaspoon honey

1. Combine the Dahi and Atasi. Stir well.

2. Add the Shatavari, Shunti, Ela, and honey. Stir until evenly blended.

3. Take after meals or as needed during acute diarrhea. For chronic loose stools, take 1 to 2 times daily until remedied.

Atisar Basti

Makes 1 application

During diarrhea (Atisar), the colon becomes overheated and inflamed. Basti (herbal enema) is a direct therapy for GI distress. This remedy uses a decoction of cooling, anti-inflammatory, and astringent herbs that soothe the membrane and bind stool. Avoid food three to four hours before and after using. This therapy is best for chronic loose stools; avoid with acute diarrhea or flare-ups. Rest, eat light, and drink lots of warm water on enema days. You can use a disposable or nondisposable enema bag for application.

4 cups water
2 teaspoons Guduchi powder
2 teaspoons Yashtimadhu powder (licorice)
1 teaspoon Shatavari powder
1 teaspoon Arjuna powder

1. In a saucepan over high heat, boil the water.

2. Reduce the heat to low and add the Guduchi, Yashtimadhu, Shatavari, and Arjuna. Steep, mostly covered, on a simmer until 2 cups liquid remain, about 60 minutes. Stir occasionally.

3. Strain and cool to body temperature.

4. Pour the decoction into an enema bag.

5. Insert the tubing and allow the decoction to flow into the colon.

6. Hold in for at least 30 minutes, if possible. Expel when needed.

7. Use weekly for mild issues or up to 3 days weekly for more severe cases.

FATIGUE

Fatigue is a common complaint with a vast array of causes. Chronic stress, mental exhaustion, physical exhaustion, nutrient deficiency, chronic infection, sluggish digestion, toxicity, sedentary lifestyle, and depression can all contribute. Vata may create depletion, Pitta may be burnt out, or Kapha may invoke heaviness. Narrow down this list and remove your specific cause(s) to find relief. Herbal support will expedite healing and bring the vitality you deserve!

Energy Rasayana

Makes 1 serving

Ghee and honey together are the ultimate Rasayana (rejuvenative). Taken with Ashwagandha and Bala, the potency increases, while Shunti and Tvak reduce heaviness. Ayurveda states that ghee and honey become toxic when taken together in equal amounts, but that refers to weight, not volume. The ghee and honey in this recipe are not equal by weight, so follow the recipe and enjoy the nectar!

1 teaspoon ghee or coconut oil
1 teaspoon honey
½ teaspoon Ashwagandha powder
½ teaspoon Bala powder
¼ teaspoon Tvak powder (cinnamon)
¼ teaspoon Shunti powder (ginger)
1 cup warm water

1. In a small bowl, blend the ghee and honey.

2. Add the Ashwagandha, Bala, Tvak, and Shunti and stir until evenly mixed.

3. Take each morning and again around 2 p.m., when Vata enters and energy depletes. Follow with the water.

Ojas Energy Balls

Makes 15 to 18 balls (1 ball per serving)

These balls serve as both an herbal remedy and a sweet treat! This recipe boosts Ojas—the force behind our energy and vitality—to reduce fatigue and stimulate energy. Almond, Ashwagandha, and Shatavari are well-known Rasayanas (rejuvenatives) for the body, mind, and libido.

1 cup finely ground raw, unsalted almonds
2 tablespoons shredded coconut
2 tablespoons Ashwagandha powder
2 tablespoons Shatavari powder
2 teaspoons Shunti powder (ginger)
2 teaspoons Tvak powder (cinnamon)
⅛ teaspoon pink Himalayan salt
⅓ cup honey
2 tablespoons ghee or coconut oil

1. In a bowl, combine the ground almonds, coconut, Ashwagandha, Shatavari, Shunti, Tvak, and salt. Stir well.

2. Add the honey and ghee. Using your hands, mix together until the ingredients are evenly combined. Wet hands if needed to avoid sticking.

3. Roll into 15 to 18 small balls. If desired, roll the outside of the balls in extra coconut.

4. Freeze for 2 hours before serving.

5. Take one ball in the morning and again at midday.

6. Freeze in an airtight container for up to 3 months.

Rasayana Churna

Makes 1 cup powder

This formula is a total system energizer using the top Rasayana (rejuvenative) herbs. It is perfect during times of mental fatigue, as well as physical exhaustion. This revitalizing synergy of herbs strengthens muscle, nourishes tissues, regenerates cells, tones nerves, and invigorates the mind. Take upon awakening and again at midday if energy begins to wane.

4 tablespoons Ashwagandha powder
4 tablespoons Bala powder
4 tablespoons Brahmi powder
4 tablespoons Guduchi powder
1 teaspoon Shunti powder (ginger)
½ cup warm water (per serving)
½ teaspoon ghee (per serving, optional)
1 teaspoon honey (per serving, optional)

1. In a small bowl, blend the Ashwagandha, Bala, Brahmi, Guduchi, and Shunti.

2. Take ½ teaspoon of herbs mixed in the water. Alternatively, mix ½ teaspoon of herbs with the ghee and honey and follow with the water.

3. Store in an airtight glass jar for up to 1 year.

FEVER

Fever (Jwara) appears frequently in ancient texts. Mild fevers may occur during a cold, while more severe fevers tend to accompany infection. Ayurveda states that fever stems from toxins invading the blood, plasma, and lymphatic system. This creates high temperatures, body aches, and lethargy while dousing Agni (digestive fire). Treat fever with a broth, fasting or light eating, hot water, ginger baths, and total rest.

Farewell Fever Tea

Makes 6 cups

Although fever increases body temperature, certain heating herbs can be helpful for treatment. Tulsi and Shunti act directly on Rasavaha Srotas, the lymphatic system, which is attacked when fever strikes. The heating energy of this trio destroys pathogens and induces sweating. Fever also douses digestion, and this tea will give your Agni (gastric fire) a spark. Eat simply and lightly until health returns.

6½ cups water
4 tablespoons cut-and-sifted Tulsi
2 tablespoons cut-and-sifted Shunti (dry ginger)
3 Tvak (cinnamon) sticks
2 tablespoons honey

1. In a large saucepan over high heat, boil the water.

2. Reduce the heat to low; add the Tulsi, Shunti, and Tvak. Steep on a simmer, mostly covered, for 20 to 30 minutes.

3. Strain and cool slightly. Stir in the honey.

4. Drink 1 cup every 1 to 2 hours during fevers over 100°F. Drink every 2 to 6 hours for milder fevers.

5. Refrigerate leftover tea for up to 5 days.

Fever Reliever Soak

Makes 3 cups

Fevers leave you feeling run-down, achy, and exhausted. This heating bath soak brings relief as you sweat away the pathogens and toxins burdening your system. This formula eases muscle soreness and body aches to bring a little comfort and relaxation to your distress.

8 tablespoons Shunti powder (ginger)
8 tablespoons Tulsi powder
1 cup baking soda
1 cup Epsom salt
10 drops essential oils (e.g., rosemary, orange, or Tulsi) per soak (optional)

1. In a small bowl, blend the Shunti and Tulsi.

2. Add the baking soda and Epsom salt. Stir evenly.

3. To use, add ½ cup to a hot bath; stir until fully dissolved. Add the essential oils, if using.

4. Soak for 20 to 30 minutes. For severe fevers, soak 1 or 2 times daily or as needed. Double the recipe if needed.

5. Store in an airtight glass jar for up to 1 year.

GAS AND BLOATING

Gas and bloating are Vata imbalances, but all body types fall prey to this universal complaint. Gas often stems from improper diet but often includes mental components such as stress or anxiety. Follow a Vata-pacifying diet by avoiding cold, raw, processed, and leftover foods. Do not overeat, and do not eat before full digestion of the previous meal. Eliminate food intolerances and follow proper food combining (e.g., eating fruit with any other food type is asking for trouble). See the Resources section (page 195) for additional Ayurvedic cookbook recommendations.

Fennel-Ajwain Tea

Makes 3 cups

Gas is uncomfortable and disruptive to your daily life. This simple remedy alleviates gas and bloating and bestows healthy digestion. Ajwain relieves Vata-type digestion (i.e., gas, bloating, colic) by regulating the five Vayus (winds) in the body and expelling excessive Air. Mishreya can calm digestive distress, and Ela brings an invigorating aroma and sweet flavor, making this tea as delicious as it is healing.

> **3½ cups water**
> **1 tablespoon whole Mishreya (fennel)**
> **1 teaspoon whole Ajwain**
> **1 teaspoon hulled whole Ela (cardamom)**
> **1 to 2 teaspoons honey (optional)**

1. In a large saucepan over high heat, boil the water.

2. Reduce the heat to low; add the Mishreya, Ajwain, and Ela. Steep on a simmer, mostly covered, for 20 minutes.

3. Strain and cool slightly. Stir in the honey, if using.

4. Drink 1 cup up to 3 times daily before meals.

5. Refrigerate leftover tea for up to 5 days.

Vata Honey

Makes 1 cup honey

When gas and bloating arise, Vata is at play. By the powerful gut-brain connection, even high Vata in the mind (e.g., anxiety, fear, hyperactivity) leads to high Vata in the colon (e.g., gas, bloating). This formula works to reduce systemic Vata while boosting digestion and relieving intestinal spasm. For long-term gas and bloating issues, take this remedy daily with each meal.

3 tablespoons Mishreya powder (fennel)
2 tablespoons Dhanya powder (coriander)
2 tablespoons Ashwagandha powder
1 teaspoon Shunti powder (ginger)
1 teaspoon Tvak powder (cinnamon)
½ teaspoon Ajwain powder
½ teaspoon Ela powder (cardamom)
1 cup honey
2 tablespoons freshly squeezed lemon juice
½ cup warm water (per serving)

1. In a small bowl, blend the Mishreya, Dhanya, Ashwagandha, Shunti, Tvak, Ajwain, and Ela.

2. Add the honey. Blend evenly.

3. Stir in the lemon juice.

4. Take 1 teaspoon 3 times daily before meals or as needed during flare-ups. Follow with the warm water.

5. Store in an airtight glass jar for up to 1 year; no refrigeration is needed.

Wind-Releasing Tincture

Makes 2 cups

This gut-soothing formula calms intestinal spasms and relieves colic (abdominal spasm). It increases the digestive force and facilitates the release of excessive Wind (Vayu) in the gastrointestinal tract. Taking this tincture before meals kindles Agni (digestion) to prevent flatulence. Tinctures should steep for at least 28 days for best potency, but it's worth the wait!

5 tablespoons Haritaki powder
5 tablespoons Mishreya powder (fennel)
3 tablespoons Ajwain powder
2 tablespoons Shunti powder (ginger)
1 tablespoon Chitrak powder
3 cups brandy or glycerin

1. In a small bowl, mix the Haritaki, Mishreya, Ajwain, Shunti, and Chitrak. Pour the mixture into a 1-quart mason jar.

2. Add the brandy or glycerin, pouring until the liquid fills just below the top of the jar. Cover and shake.

3. Let sit for 28 days. Shake every 1 to 3 days.

4. Using a fine-mesh strainer covered with muslin cloth, strain the herbs. To get more yield, use your hands to carefully squeeze out excess liquid.

5. Fill a small glass dropper bottle for daily use. Take 3 to 10 droppers full 3 times daily before meals, or as needed during flare-ups.

6. Store tincture in a glass jar for up to 3 years for brandy-based extract and up to 2 years for glycerin-based extract.

HAIR CARE

Poor hair health can reveal internal imbalances. In Ayurveda, hair loss and premature graying indicate elevated Pitta "burning" hair at its follicles. Because hair is a by-product of bones (Asthi dhatu), brittle hair may signify brittle bones. Other negative influences include stress, insomnia, hormonal imbalance, thyroid disorder, deficiency, and depletion. Encourage healthy hair with a wholesome diet, nightly scalp massages, deep breathing, and inverted yoga postures such as "legs up the wall" or shoulder stand.

Clarifying Hair Rinse

Makes 4 cups

Apple cider vinegar is a hair care tonic. It removes dullness, strengthens strands, alleviates dandruff, and eliminates fungus and bacteria that may attack the scalp. Amalaki and Bhringaraj are healthy hair powerhouses, boosting growth and regeneration. This infusion process takes 14 days for steeping.

5 tablespoons Amalaki powder
5 tablespoons Bhringaraj powder
3 tablespoons Bibhitaki powder
3 tablespoons Haritaki powder
5 cups apple cider vinegar
1 cup warm water (per use)

1. In a small bowl, mix the Amalaki, Bhringaraj, Bibhitaki, and Haritaki. Transfer to a 1-quart mason jar.

2. Add the apple cider vinegar, pouring until the liquid fills just below the top of the jar. Cover and shake.

3. Let the jar sit for 14 days. Shake every 1 to 2 days.

4. Using a fine-mesh strainer covered with muslin cloth, strain the herbs.

5. To use, add 2 to 4 tablespoons to 1 cup of warm water. After shampooing and conditioning, apply mixture to scalp and hair. Let sit for 5 minutes, then rinse.

6. Store in an airtight glass jar for up to 1 year.

Hair Care Churna

Makes 1 cup powder

Healthy hair is rooted from the inside out. These three herbs are leaders in Ayurvedic hair care for internal and external uses. Together, they stimulate hair growth, prevent graying, and provide antioxidants for regeneration. For most noticeable results, take this formula daily while using the Clarifying Hair Rinse (page 152) and Bhringaraj Hair Oil (page 61) weekly.

8 tablespoons Bhringaraj powder
5 tablespoons Brahmi powder
3 tablespoons Amalaki powder
1 cup warm water (per serving)

1. In a small bowl, blend the Bhringaraj, Brahmi, and Amalaki.

2. Add 1 teaspoon of powder to the water. Take upon awakening and before bed. Use consistently for best results.

3. Store the herbs in an airtight glass jar for up to 1 year.

HEADACHE

Headache is called *Shira Shula* in Sanskrit. Ayurveda states that there is no pain without stagnation. This rings true, as headaches are often caused by constriction (Vata), inflammation (Pitta), or congestion (Kapha), resulting in limited circulation and oxygen going to the head. The specific causes of headaches are vast and are different for each individual. Some universal therapies include ginger baths; head, neck, and shoulder massage; deep breathing; meditation; and relaxation.

Headache Relief Tea

Makes 4 cups

Headaches can stem from many causes, but encouraging circulation to the brain can bring universal relief. This tea's spicy nature clears congestion, stimulates blood flow, and relieves pain. Brahmi and Ardraka relieve stress, another common factor. Sit with the tea, breathe deep, and calm the mind.

4½ cups water
1 (2-inch) cube (20 grams) Ardraka (fresh ginger), finely minced
1 teaspoon freshly ground Sarshapa (brown mustard seed)
1 teaspoon freshly ground Maricha (black pepper)
2 tablespoons cut-and-sifted Brahmi
1 tablespoon honey (optional)

1. In a large saucepan, boil the water.

2. Reduce the heat to low; add the Ardraka, Sarshapa, Maricha, and Brahmi. Steep on a low simmer for 20 minutes.

3. Strain and cool slightly. Stir in the honey, if using.

4. Drink 1 cup every 2 hours at the first sign of headache, or as needed.

5. Refrigerate leftover tea for up to 5 days.

Headache Relief Oil

Makes 4 cups

This oil is essential for anyone experiencing frequent headaches or migraines. These heating herbs reduce pain and inflammation while promoting circulation. Massage the oil onto the forehead, scalp, and feet nightly for headache prevention, or apply after onset. For severe symptoms, soak a cloth in the oil and place it on the forehead for at least 20 minutes. This oil takes three days to prepare.

5 cups sesame oil
6 tablespoons Brahmi powder
3 tablespoons Shunti powder (ginger)
3 tablespoons Sarshapa powder (brown mustard seed)
2 tablespoons Tvak powder (cinnamon)
2 tablespoons Lavanga powder (clove)

1. Preheat the oven to 175°F.

2. In an oven-safe baking dish, stir the oil, Brahmi, Shunti, Sarshapa, Tvak, and Lavanga to combine.

3. Place the baking dish, uncovered, in the oven. Heat for 8 hours, stirring every 2 to 4 hours.

4. Let the baking dish sit for 12 hours in the oven with the heat off.

5. Remove the baking dish, stir well, and repeat steps 3 and 4 twice, preheating the oven again each time. This process takes 3 days total.

6. Using a fine-mesh strainer covered with muslin cloth, strain the herbs from the oil. To get more yield, use your hands to squeeze out excess oil.

7. Pour the oil into a bottle or jar.

8. Store for up to 1 year.

Brahmi-Ghee Nasya

Makes 1 cup

Nasya is the administration of herbal medicine through the nose. It acts directly on the mind for stress reduction and headache relief. Although tridoshic (balances all doshas), Brahmi Ghee is best for Pitta-induced headaches stemming from heat, inflammation, acidity, anger, or stress. It is gentle enough for daily use but can be used symptomatically as well. This remedy takes three days to prepare.

1 cup ghee, melted
¼ cup Brahmi powder

1. Preheat the oven to 175°F.

2. In an oven-safe baking dish, stir the ghee and Brahmi to combine.

3. Place the baking dish, uncovered, in the oven. Heat for 8 hours, stirring every 2 to 4 hours.

4. Let the baking dish sit for 12 hours in the oven with the heat off.

5. Remove the baking dish, stir, and repeat steps 3 and 4 twice, preheating the oven again each time. This process takes 3 days total.

6. Using a fine-mesh strainer covered with muslin cloth, strain the herbs from the ghee. To get more yield, use your hands to squeeze out excess ghee.

7. Fill a glass dropper bottle for daily use.

8. Apply 1 to 5 drops of ghee into each nostril upon awakening. If the ghee solidifies, soak the closed bottle in warm water. Apply as needed for acute headaches, or use daily for ongoing care.

HIGH CHOLESTEROL

High cholesterol results from excessive Kapha accumulating in the blood. It may stem from heavy diet, sedentary living, weak liver, thyroid imbalance, obesity, genetics, or medications. Generally, high cholesterol can be controlled by diet, lifestyle, herbs—and discipline! A Kapha-reducing diet limiting refined carbs, unhealthy fats, red meat, pork, and dairy is essential. Exercise for at least 30 minutes daily and use your herbal remedies consistently for best results.

Cinnamon Honey Plus

Makes 1 cup

This morning remedy supplements a healthy diet and lifestyle for reducing cholesterol naturally. It accelerates the magic of Tvak and honey with additional help from the "three pungents" of Trikatu. This spicy combo encourages healthy digestion and metabolism, and lower cholesterol levels.

½ teaspoon Tvak powder (cinnamon)
¼ teaspoon Shunti powder (ginger)
⅛ teaspoon Maricha powder (black pepper)
⅛ teaspoon Pippali powder
1 teaspoon honey
1 cup warm water

1. In a small bowl, blend the Tvak, Shunti, Maricha, and Pippali.

2. Add the honey and stir until evenly mixed.

3. Take each morning, following with the water. For severe issues, repeat dosage before bed.

Cholesterol Care Churna

Makes 1 cup powder

No heart health program is complete without Arjuna! It strengthens the heart while reducing Kapha (cholesterol) in the blood. Guggulu stimulates metabolism and works to scrape fat and cholesterol from the system. Shunti and Chitrak ignite Agni (digestive fire) to prevent future cholesterol accumulation. Take daily with a Kapha-reducing diet and exercise program for a healthier heart.

6 tablespoons Guggulu powder
4 tablespoons Arjuna powder
3 tablespoons Shunti powder (ginger)
3 tablespoons Chitrak powder
1 cup warm water (per serving)

1. In a small bowl, blend the Guggulu, Arjuna, Shunti, and Chitrak.

2. Combine 1 teaspoon of powder with the water. Take upon awakening and repeat before bed. Be consistent for best results.

3. Store the herbs in an airtight glass jar for up to 1 year.

HYPERACIDITY

Hyperacidity (Amlapitta) is connected to Pitta dosha and Annavaha Srotas (gastrointestinal tract). Proton-pump inhibitors are often prescribed, but can create dependency and lead to negative side effects. Hyperacidity can often be controlled naturally with diet and lifestyle changes. Follow a Pitta-reducing diet by avoiding hot, spicy, acidic, oily, and fermented foods. Eat light dinners before 6 p.m., go for walks, and keep stress and anger low!

Everyday Antacid

Makes 1 cup powder

This soothing formula is a holistic antacid for prevention or symptom relief. Hyperacidity means high Pitta in the gastrointestinal tract. This herbal trio calms Pitta in the gut to reduce heat, absorb excessive acids, soothe inflammation, and heal the mucosal membrane. For chronic heartburn or reflux, take before meals daily until long-term relief is established.

6 tablespoons Shatavari powder
5 tablespoons Guduchi powder
5 tablespoons Yashtimadhu powder (licorice)
½ cup warm water (per serving)

1. In a small bowl, blend the Shatavari, Guduchi, and Yashtimadhu.

2. Combine 1 teaspoon of powder with the water and take as needed. For chronic issues, take ½ teaspoon with the water 3 times daily before meals.

3. Store the herbs in an airtight glass jar in a dry, cool, dark environment for up to 1 year.

Acid-Reducing Tonic

Makes 1 cup

Baking soda boasts an alkaline pH to neutralize acidity in the gut. When taken with lime juice, the chemical reaction creates a fizziness to calm stomach woes. Amalaki, Shunti, and Ela help out by decreasing heat (Pitta) in the gastrointestinal tract and soothing the gut lining. If you have recurring hyperacidity issues, keep this Ayurvedic-friendly remedy on hand.

¼ **teaspoon Amalaki powder**
⅛ **teaspoon Shunti powder (ginger)**
¼ **teaspoon Ela powder (cardamom)**
1 cup warm water
Juice of ½ lime
½ **teaspoon baking soda**

1. Combine the Amalaki, Shunti, Ela, and water.

2. Add the lime juice. Stir well.

3. Just before taking, stir in the baking soda.

4. Drink by sipping, not gulping. The bubbles may create gas if taken too quickly.

5. Drink anytime heartburn, hyperacidity, reflux, or "sour stomach" arises.

HYPERGLYCEMIA

Hyperglycemia (high blood sugar) results from insufficient insulin and is often associated with diabetes (Prameha). Ancient texts list 20 different types of Prameha, each with specific symptoms and treatments. Whether you are diabetic, prediabetic, or simply at risk, follow a Kapha-reducing diet, avoiding sweets, refined carbs, overeating, and eating past 6 p.m. Don't forget to exercise! If you are on blood sugar medication, use remedies under a physician's guidance.

Blood Sugar Balance Churna

Makes 1 cup powder

Bitter is better for a healthy pancreas and blood sugar levels. With only two herbal ingredients, this remedy acts directly on the pancreas and liver, two key players in hyperglycemia conditions. It strengthens, cleanses, and cools these vital organs, facilitating the absorption of glucose to help balance blood sugar levels.

8 tablespoons Haridra powder
8 tablespoons Neem powder
½ cup warm water (per serving)

1. In a small bowl, blend the Haridra and Neem.

2. Combine ½ teaspoon of powder with the water. Take 3 times daily before meals. Be consistent for best results.

3. Store the herbs in an airtight glass jar in a dry, cool, dark environment for up to 1 year.

Tulsi-Cinnamon Support Tea

Makes 6 cups

This sweet, simple tea recipe supports healthy blood sugar levels. Tulsi improves pancreatic functioning and stimulates insulin secretion. Tvak reduces insulin resistance to encourage lower blood glucose levels. This mighty duo stimulates digestion and removes excessive Kapha, two common issues with high blood sugar conditions.

6½ cups water
5 tablespoons cut-and-sifted Tulsi
3 Tvak (cinnamon) sticks

1. In a large saucepan, boil the water.

2. Reduce the heat to low; add the Tulsi and Tvak. Steep on a low simmer, mostly covered, for 20 to 30 minutes. Strain.

3. Drink 1 cup 1 to 3 times daily, before meals.

4. Refrigerate leftover tea for up to 5 days.

HYPERTENSION

Hypertension (high blood pressure), or Sirabhinodhana, has three main types: Vata-type, associated with anxiety, worry, and fear; Pitta-type, involving anger, stress, and excessive heat; and Kapha-type, resulting from high triglycerides, high cholesterol, excessive weight, and sedentary living. Match your diet and lifestyle to your hypertension type to support balance and use meditation and relaxation to complement all treatments.

Blood Pressure Support Tincture

Makes 2 cups

Hypertension has various causes, making it necessary to combat it from different angles. Arjuna strengthens the heart, Punarnava and Kalmegha reduce congestion, and Bhring-haraj and Shankapushpi calm stress. If you are on blood pressure medication, use under a physician's guidance. This tincture recipe takes 28 days for full extraction.

4 tablespoons Arjuna powder	3 tablespoons Shankapushpi powder
3 tablespoons Punarnava powder	3 tablespoons Kalmegha powder
3 tablespoons Bhringaraj powder	3 cups brandy or glycerin

1. In a small bowl, mix the Arjuna, Punarnava, Bhringaraj, Shankapushpi, and Kalmegha.

2. Combine the herbs in a 1-quart mason jar. Add the brandy or glycerin, pouring until the liquid fills just below the top of the jar; cover and shake.

3. Let the jar sit for 28 days. Shake every 3 days.

4. Using a fine-mesh strainer covered with muslin cloth, strain the herbs from the brandy or glycerin. To get more yield, use your hands to carefully squeeze out excess liquid.

5. Fill a small glass dropper bottle for daily use. Take 3 to 6 droppers full 3 times daily after meals.

6. Store tincture in a glass jar for up to 3 years for brandy-based extract and up to 2 years for glycerin-based extract.

Healthy Blood Pressure Churna

Makes 1 cup powder

This formula helps alleviate high blood pressure naturally. These herbs work in harmony to reduce stress and tension, clear channels (srotamsi), and reduce inflammation. Take this remedy mixed in CCF and Ardraka Tea (page 165) as a carrier to enhance its diuretic properties and further reduce blood pressure, or simply take in warm water. Whatever your method, consistency is key! If you are on blood pressure medication, use only under a physician's guidance.

> **5 tablespoons Shankapushpi powder**
> **5 tablespoons Punarnava powder**
> **3 tablespoons Arjuna powder**
> **3 tablespoons Bhringaraj powder**
> **1 tablespoon Haridra powder (turmeric)**
> **1 cup CCF and Ardraka Tea (page 165) or warm water (per serving)**

1. In a small bowl, blend the Shankapushpi, Punarnava, Arjuna, Bhringaraj, and Haridra.

2. Add ½ to 1 teaspoon to the tea or water. Take upon awakening and again before bed.

3. Store the herbs in an airtight glass jar in a dry, cool, dark environment for up to 1 year.

INDIGESTION

Indigestion (Ajirna) relates to Manda Agni, the Kapha digestion type. Symptoms include dull appetite, undue fullness, and nausea. If there is heartburn or acidity, Pitta is involved as well. Weak digestion is said to be the root cause of all disease. We must digest our food well to prevent illness and maintain health. Kitchari cleanses or intermittent fasting help reset the Agni (digestive fire). Follow a Kapha-reducing diet and avoid overeating, snacking, heavy foods, and eating after 6 p.m.

CCF and Ardraka Tea

Makes 6 cups

CCF and Ardraka Tea is adapted from a well-known recipe taught by Dr. Vasant Lad. This simple remedy is suitable for all body types and is gentle enough for daily use. These common spices kindle Agni (digestive fire), flush toxins (Ama), and alleviate indigestion. A main cause of toxicity is undigested food. Drinking this tea between meals allows your body to process food and prepare you for future meals.

6½ cups water
2 tablespoons whole Mishreya (fennel)
2 tablespoons whole Dhanya (coriander)
1 tablespoon whole Jirak (cumin)
2 tablespoons grated Ardraka (fresh ginger)

1. In a large saucepan, boil the water.

2. Reduce the heat to low. Add the Mishreya, Dhanya, Jirak, and Ardraka.

3. Steep on a low simmer, mostly covered, for 20 to 30 minutes. Strain.

4. Drink 1 cup 1 to 3 times daily upon awakening and between meals.

5. Refrigerate leftover tea for up to 5 days.

Healthy Digestion Honey

Makes 1 cup

Indigestion is often a sign of sluggish digestion known as Manda Agni (slow fire). This weakened state of digestion creates toxicity, slow metabolism, weight gain, congestion, and lethargy. This heating honey will stimulate your fire (Agni) and get things cooking. Healthy digestion brings lightness, energy, and well-being, and this remedy will help you achieve that!

3 tablespoons Mishreya powder (fennel)
2 tablespoons Haridra powder (turmeric)
2 tablespoons Shunti powder (ginger)
1 tablespoon Tvak powder (cinnamon)
1 tablespoon Chitrak powder
1 teaspoon Maricha powder (black pepper)
1 cup honey
2 tablespoons freshly squeezed lemon juice

1. In a small bowl, blend the Mishreya, Haridra, Shunti, Tvak, Chitrak, and Maricha.

2. Add the honey and blend evenly.

3. Stir in the lemon juice.

4. Take 1 teaspoon 3 times daily, directly before meals. Follow with a few sips of warm water. Be consistent for best results!

5. Store in an airtight glass jar for up to 1 year; no refrigeration is needed.

Digestive Tonic Tincture

Makes 2 cups

This tincture provides quick relief for digestive distress. It penetrates the gastrointestinal tract to ignite Agni (digestion), spark metabolism, burn toxins, and relieve indigestion. Tinctures are easy to take on the go! Keep a bottle at home, at work, and when traveling. Take before meals for prevention or as needed for prompt care. This remedy requires a 28-day steep for total extraction.

5 tablespoons Guduchi powder
3 tablespoons Chitrak powder
3 tablespoons Musta powder
3 tablespoons Shunti powder (ginger)
1 tablespoon Haridra powder (turmeric)
1 tablespoon Ajwain powder
3 cups brandy or glycerin

1. In a small bowl, mix the Guduchi, Chitrak, Musta, Shunti, Haridra, and Ajwain.

2. Transfer the herbs to a 1-quart mason jar. Add the brandy or glycerin, pouring until the liquid fills just below the top of the jar. Cover and shake.

3. Let the jar sit for 28 days. Shake every 3 days.

4. Using a fine-mesh strainer covered with muslin cloth, strain the herbs from the brandy or glycerin. Use your hands to squeeze out excess liquid.

5. Fill a small glass dropper bottle for daily use. Take 3 to 5 droppers full before meals or up to 7 droppers for acute indigestion.

6. Store tincture in a glass jar for up to 3 years for brandy-based extract and up to 2 years for glycerin-based extract.

INSOMNIA

Insomnia stems from Vata invading the nervous system. There is often a mental factor involved, such as anxiety, stress, or depression. Although insomnia sparks at night, examine all your living habits to find balance. Establish a stable daily routine and meal schedule, avoid caffeine and naps, exercise, limit electronics, and end work by 5 p.m. (if possible!). Use calming nighttime practices such as warm baths, foot massage, restorative yoga, and meditation to ease you into sleep.

Sleepy Tea Kshirpak

Makes 1 cup

Sleep disturbances are disruptive to your life and health. This medicated milk (kshirpak) recipe tones the nervous system to promote restful sleep. These herbs calm Vata, subdue restlessness, reduce stress, and relax nerves. Steeping slowly in milk enhances their properties for greater benefit.

1 cup milk or almond milk
1 cup water
½ teaspoon Ashwagandha powder

¼ teaspoon Shankapushpi powder
¼ teaspoon Tulsi powder
1 to 2 teaspoons honey (optional)

1. In a large saucepan over high heat, boil the milk and water.

2. Reduce the heat to low. Stir in the Ashwagandha, Shankapushpi, and Tulsi.

3. Steep on a low simmer, mostly covered, until 1 cup of milk remains. Stir every 1 to 2 minutes.

4. Let cool slightly. Stir in the honey, if using.

5. Drink 30 minutes before your desired bedtime.

Sleep Easy Oil

Makes 4 cups

Insomnia reveals imbalance in the nervous system. Abhyanga (oil massage) is a direct method for calming the nerves and promoting sound sleep. This can be self-administered, before bed, and the oil should be left on overnight. For nights when full-body massages are not in your stars, simply massage your head, neck, and feet. This oil remedy takes three days for full infusion.

> 5 cups sesame oil
> 4 tablespoons Shankapushpi powder
> 4 tablespoons Ashwagandha powder
> 3 tablespoons Brahmi powder
> 3 tablespoons Tulsi powder
> 2 tablespoons Yashtimadhu powder (licorice)
> 10 to 20 drops each lavender, rosemary, and chamomile
>   essential oils (optional)

1. Preheat the oven to 175°F.

2. In an oven-safe baking dish, stir the sesame oil, Shankapushpi, Ashwagandha, Brahmi, Tulsi, and Yashtimadhu to combine.

3. Place the baking dish, uncovered, in the oven. Heat for 8 hours, stirring every 2 to 4 hours.

4. Let the baking dish sit for 12 hours in the oven with the heat off.

5. Remove the baking dish, stir well, and repeat steps 3 and 4 twice, preheating the oven again each time. This process takes 3 days total.

6. Using a fine-mesh strainer covered with muslin cloth, strain the herbs from the oil. To get more yield, use your hands to carefully squeeze out excess oil.

7. Pour the strained oil into a bottle or jar. Stir in the lavender, rosemary, and chamomile oils (if using).

8. Store for up to 1 year.

Sweet Dreams Churna

Makes 1 cup powder

Over-the-counter sleep aids create poor sleep quality, grogginess, and dependency. This herbal formula is safe for long-term use without causing dependence. Rather than masking symptoms, these herbs decrease imbalance by strengthening the nervous system. Take 30 minutes before bed for more restful sleep. If your trouble is staying asleep, keep a premade dose in water by your bed.

6 tablespoons Ashwagandha powder
5 tablespoons Shankapushpi powder
3 tablespoons Tulsi powder
2 tablespoons Yashtimadhu powder
1 teaspoon Pippali powder
1 cup warm milk or water (per serving)
½ teaspoon ghee (per serving, optional)

1. In a small bowl, blend the Ashwagandha, Shankapushpi, Tulsi, Yashtimadhu, and Pippali.

2. Add ½ to 1 teaspoon to the warm milk or water (for best results).

3. Add the ghee, if using.

4. Store the herbs in an airtight glass jar for up to 1 year.

LOW LIBIDO

Low libido is common for people of all ages. Sex can be a healthy release and a way to keep intimacy in a relationship. A diminished sex drive often indicates low Ojas, the energetic force behind vitality, strength, and immunity. This can result from excessive stress, toxicity, overwork, exhaustion, emotional imbalance, or relationship issues. Nourishing Ojas, cleansing, and balancing the mind are helpful tools for sparking sexual potency!

Ojas Milk

Makes 1 cup

Low libido is not a natural occurrence, but a sign of imbalance. This formula builds Ojas and revitalizes libido. Ashwagandha, Shatavari, Bala, and Keshar strengthen reproductive organs and soothe stress. Shunti and Ela provide warmth and stimulate circulation. Milk, ghee, and honey are the rejuvenative catalysts that complete this aphrodisiac drink. Avoid with high Kapha or signs of high toxins, including heavy tongue coating, sluggish digestion, and congestion.

1 cup milk or almond milk
¼ cup water
½ teaspoon Ashwagandha powder
½ teaspoon Shatavari powder
¼ teaspoon Bala powder

¼ teaspoon Shunti powder (ginger)
⅛ teaspoon Ela powder (cardamom)
3 Keshar threads (saffron)
1 teaspoon ghee
1 teaspoon honey

1. In a large saucepan over high heat, boil the milk and water.

2. Reduce the heat to low. Add the Ashwagandha, Shatavari, Bala, Shunti, Ela, Keshar, and ghee. Steep on a low simmer for 5 minutes, stirring every 30 to 45 seconds.

3. Cool slightly. Stir in the honey.

4. Drink 30 minutes before intercourse, or take 2 to 4 times weekly for ongoing support.

Aphrodisiac Almond-Date Shake

Makes 1 serving

This delicious drink increases Ojas (vitality), enhances energy, and stimulates libido. Take it as a light breakfast or midday snack to revitalize sexual potency. This drink is sweet and heavy by nature; limit to three times weekly to avoid congestion. Kapha types should omit ghee, replace dates with 1½ teaspoons of honey, and double the Tvak and Shunti. Avoid altogether when experiencing signs of high toxins, including heavy tongue coating, sluggish digestion, and congestion.

3 Khajoor (dates), pitted and chopped
1½ cups water
15 almonds, soaked and peeled
½ teaspoon Ashwagandha powder
½ teaspoon Shatavari powder
¼ teaspoon Shunti powder (ginger)
¼ teaspoon Tvak powder (cinnamon)
⅛ teaspoon Ela powder (cardamom)
3 Keshar threads (saffron)
1 teaspoon ghee

1. Soak the Khajoor in the water for 30 minutes, or until soft.

2. Place the almonds and dates with their soaking water into a blender.

3. Add the Ashwagandha, Shatavari, Shunti, Tvak, Ela, Keshar, and ghee.

4. Blend on high for 3 minutes, or until smooth.

Aphrodisiac Oil

Makes 4 cups

Aphrodisiac Oil warms the body and gets the blood flowing. Use it to massage the pelvic region and genitals to encourage circulation. Men experiencing impotency and premature ejaculation will find benefit through daily massage. Women experiencing dryness and diminished libido should apply routinely. This medicated oil also serves as a natural lubricant! This recipe requires three days of steeping time.

5 cups sesame oil
4 tablespoons Ashwagandha powder
4 tablespoons Shatavari powder
3 tablespoons Bala powder
3 tablespoons Shunti powder (ginger)
2 tablespoons Tvak powder (cinnamon)

20 Keshar threads (saffron)
20 drops rosemary essential oil (optional)
20 drops cedarwood essential oil (optional)
5 drops ginger essential oil (optional)

1. Preheat the oven to 175°F.

2. In an oven-safe baking dish, stir the sesame oil, Ashwagandha, Shatavari, Bala, Shunti, Tvak, and Keshar to combine.

3. Place the baking dish, uncovered, in the oven. Heat for 8 hours, stirring every 2 to 4 hours.

4. Let the baking dish sit for 12 hours in the oven with the heat off.

5. Remove the baking dish, stir, and repeat steps 3 and 4 twice, preheating the oven again each time. This process takes 3 days total.

6. Using a fine-mesh strainer covered with muslin cloth, strain the herbs from the oil. To get more yield, use your hands to carefully squeeze out excess oil.

7. Transfer the strained oil to a bottle or jar. Stir in the rosemary, cedarwood, and ginger essential oils, if using.

8. Store for up to 1 year.

MEMORY

Memory naturally wanes as we age, but severe memory issues are not inevitable. Poor memory may stem from high Vata creating constricted blood flow, poor sleep, restless thinking, or spaciness. Alternatively, high Kapha may induce congested blood flow, mental dullness, heaviness, and fogginess. Treatment varies depending on the dosha involved. However, inverted yoga postures, deep belly breathing, detoxification, increasing digestion, and head and neck massage are universal remedies.

Memory Milk

Makes 1 cup

To keep memory strong as we age, we must do what we can before it pervasively declines. Brahmi is key for supporting clarity, sharpness, and memory. Whether for treatment or prevention, this medicated milk enhances mental functioning and preserves mental vitality. Milk and ghee improve absorption, Shunti enhances potency, and a touch of Ela aids digestion. For high Kapha (congestion, excess weight) or signs of high toxins (tongue coating), replace the milk with ½ cup almond milk and ½ cup water.

1 cup milk or almond milk
¼ cup water
½ teaspoon Brahmi powder
¼ teaspoon Shunti powder (ginger)

⅛ teaspoon Ela powder (cardamom)
½ teaspoon ghee or coconut oil
1 teaspoon honey

1. In a large saucepan over high heat, boil the milk and water.

2. Reduce the heat to low. Add the Brahmi, Shunti, Ela, and ghee. Steep on a low simmer, mostly covered, for 5 minutes. Stir every 30 to 45 seconds.

3. Cool slightly. Stir in the honey.

4. Drink 30 minutes before bed.

Medhya Rasayana Churna

Makes 1 cup powder

Medhya Rasayana is a classical group of herbs that helps improve mental functioning and prevent mental decline. Of this group, these four herbs are considered the masters. Although this churna (powder) can be taken in warm water, its powers are magnified with a lipid source for direct absorption into the brain, so ghee can be very helpful here. This formula stimulates memory best when taken daily, so don't forget!

5 tablespoons Shankapushpi powder
5 tablespoons Brahmi powder
5 tablespoons Guduchi powder
2 tablespoons Yashtimadhu powder
1 cup warm milk, almond milk, or water (per serving)
½ teaspoon ghee (per serving)
1 teaspoon honey (per serving)

1. In a small bowl, blend the Shankapushpi, Brahmi, Guduchi, and Yashtimadhu.

2. Add ¾ teaspoon of herbs to the milk.

3. Add the ghee and honey.

4. Take upon awakening and before bed.

5. Store the herbs in an airtight glass jar for up to 1 year.

Medhya Nasya

Makes 1 cup

This nasya (nasal oil) awakens memory, focus, and clarity, and prevents mental deterioration. Administering Medhya (mind tonic) herbs through the nasal cavity stimulates the mind. This remedy can be done alongside Medhya Rasayana Churna (page 175) for enhanced benefits. This remedy takes three days for full steeping time.

1 cup sesame oil
1½ tablespoons Brahmi powder
1 tablespoon Shankapushpi powder
1 tablespoon Guduchi powder
1½ teaspoons Yashtimadhu powder (licorice)

1. Preheat the oven to 175°F.

2. In an oven-safe baking dish, stir the oil, Brahmi, Shankapushpi, Guduchi, and Yashtimadhu to combine.

3. Place the baking dish, uncovered, in the oven. Heat for 8 hours, stirring every 2 to 4 hours.

4. Let the baking dish sit for 12 hours in the oven with the heat off.

5. Remove the baking dish, stir, and repeat steps 3 and 4 twice, preheating the oven again each time. This process takes 3 days total.

6. Using a fine-mesh strainer covered with muslin cloth, strain the herbs from the oil. Use your hands to squeeze out excess oil.

7. Fill a glass dropper bottle for daily use. Apply 1 to 5 drops of oil into each nostril upon awakening.

8. Store extra in an airtight glass jar for up to 1 year.

ORAL CARE

The mouth is an intricate part of our microbiome. It is the origin of three srotamsi (channels): food, water, and respiratory. Maintaining our teeth, gums, and tongue is essential for total health. Scraping the tongue, using a natural toothpaste or powder, flossing, and oil-pulling are essential parts of a healthy oral routine.

Herbal Tooth Powder

Makes 1 cup

Herbal tooth powders have been gaining recent popularity. Many toothpastes contain harsh ingredients and unhealthy additives. Tooth powders are safe, effective, and gentle for daily use. This formula provides protection from receding gums, gingivitis, bad breath, mouth sores, pain, and inflammation. For daily care and freshness, scrape the tongue, brush with tooth powder, and complete with oil-pulling using Gandusha Oil (page 178).

6 tablespoons Guduchi powder
3 tablespoons Bhringaraj powder
3 tablespoons Amalaki powder
½ teaspoon Tvak powder (cinnamon)

2 tablespoons Yashtimadhu powder (licorice)
½ teaspoon Lavanga powder (clove)
½ teaspoon Neem powder
¼ teaspoon coconut oil (per serving)

1. In a small bowl, blend the Guduchi, Bhringaraj, Amalaki, Tvak, Yashtimadhu, Lavanga, and Neem.

2. Transfer ⅛ to ¼ teaspoon of herbs to a second bowl and add the water or oil to make a paste.

3. Apply to a toothbrush. Brush the teeth gently for at least 1 minute. Rinse with warm water.

4. Store the herbs in an airtight glass jar for up to 1 year.

Gandusha Oil

Makes 4 cups

Gandusha is the ancient practice of oil-pulling. This mouth oil supports oral health by strengthening gums, reducing inflammation, preventing cavities, eliminating gingivitis, and freshening breath. This recipe takes three days to prepare.

4 cups sesame oil

1 cup coconut oil

4 tablespoons Guduchi powder

4 tablespoons Bala powder

4 tablespoons Amalaki powder

2 tablespoons Musta powder

2 tablespoons Yashtimadhu powder (licorice)

1 teaspoon Neem powder

40 drops peppermint essential oil (optional)

8 drops fennel essential oil (optional)

5 drops clove essential oil (optional)

1. Preheat the oven to 175°F.

2. In an oven-safe baking dish, stir the sesame oil, coconut oil, Guduchi, Bala, Amalaki, Musta, Yashtimadhu, and Neem to combine.

3. Place the baking dish, uncovered, in the oven. Heat for 8 hours, stirring every 2 to 4 hours.

4. Let the baking dish sit for 12 hours in the oven with the heat off.

5. Remove the baking dish, stir, and repeat steps 3 and 4 twice, preheating the oven again each time. This process takes 3 days total.

6. Using a strainer covered with muslin cloth, strain the herbs. Use your hands to squeeze out excess oil.

7. Pour the oil into a bottle or jar. Stir in the peppermint, fennel, and clove oils, if using.

8. After cleaning the mouth, swish 2 tablespoons for 5 to 20 minutes; spit out. Perform daily.

9. Store the oil for up to 1 year.

PARASITIC INFECTION

Ayurveda is the foremost leader in treating Krumi, or parasitic infection. Because the root cause is weak digestion, treatment involves eliminating infection while sparking digestion (Agni) and burning toxins (Ama). Along with herbal remedies, following an antiparasitic diet and getting lots of rest is crucial. Die-off reactions may bring flu-like symptoms, making a slow, steady protocol a much smoother route.

7-Day Vidanga Cleanse

Makes 1 serving

This potent remedy is intended for strong individuals not sensitive to herbs. A strong dose of Vidanga attacks parasites effectively, and castor oil works as a purgative to flush away die-off. If you tend toward constipation, use 2 tablespoons of castor oil rather than one. Be prepared for a strong flush of the colon in the morning! Follow cleanse with ongoing Parasite-Cleansing Churna (page 180).

1 teaspoon Vidanga
1 cup warm water
1 to 2 tablespoons organic castor oil (for 7th day only)

1. Combine the Vidanga with the water.

2. Drink each night before bed for 7 nights.

3. On the seventh night, add the castor oil.

Precautions: Avoid in pregnancy or while trying to conceive (for all people). Use cautiously while experiencing hyperacidity, diarrhea, or loose stools. Discontinue use if any sensitivity reactions (rash, heat, pain, etc.) occur.

Parasite-Cleansing Churna

Makes 1 cup powder

This potent blend is a great complement for parasite cleanses, but it is also suitable for daily use. This bitter formula attacks worms, parasites, and candidiasis and supports a natural, cleansing, detoxifying process in the body. For daily use, take as suggested for a maximum of 30 to 90 days. For intense cleanses, temporarily double the dose.

5 tablespoons Guduchi powder

5 tablespoons Vidanga powder

2 tablespoons Musta powder

2 tablespoons Kalmegha powder

2 tablespoons Chitrak powder

½ cup warm water (per serving)

1. In a small bowl, blend the Guduchi, Vidanga, Musta, Kalmegha, and Chitrak.

2. Add ½ teaspoon of powder to the water. Take 3 times daily before meals. Be consistent for best results.

3. Store the herbs in an airtight glass jar in a dry, cool, dark environment for up to 1 year.

SKIN CARE

Healthy skin comes from the inside out. Many skin disorders stem from high Pitta, heat, and toxicity in the liver and blood. Cooling and cleansing these tissues will lead to healthier, clearer skin. Food allergens, hormonal imbalance, stress, poor sleep, poor diet, and unhealthy living habits may be involved as well. Combining an internal skin-supportive formula with an appropriate topical treatment is the most efficient approach to having healthy skin.

Triphala Face Mask

Makes 1 application

This face mask combines the powers of Triphala with a nourishing base oil for a clean, soft, and luminous complexion. These herbs boast significant antioxidant properties to reduce aging and clarify skin. Use coconut oil for oily, sensitive, or acne-prone skin; use sesame oil for dry, scaly, flaky skin. If you are a little of both, try combining the two.

> **2 teaspoons Amalaki powder**
> **1½ teaspoons Haritaki powder**
> **1½ teaspoons Bibhitaki powder**
> **3 tablespoons melted coconut oil or sesame oil**

1. In a small bowl, combine the Amalaki, Haritaki, and Bibhitaki. Add the oil and stir.

2. Transfer the mixture to an airtight glass jar.

3. To use, slowly massage a thin layer onto clean, dry facial skin. Massage well to stimulate circulation and exfoliation.

4. Keep on for at least 15 minutes; rinse off with warm water (no soap!).

5. Apply 1 to 3 times a week.

6. Store extra in a dry, cool place for up to 1 year.

Healthy Skin Oil

Makes 4 cups

This remedy soothes inflammation and leaves skin soft, alleviating skin conditions such as eczema, psoriasis, dermatitis, rash, cracking, and dryness. Massage onto affected areas or use as an Abhyanga (massage) oil for a total body treat! This oil takes three days for full infusion.

  4 cups sesame oil
  1 cup castor oil
  5 tablespoons Neem powder
  4 tablespoons Guduchi powder
  3 tablespoons Bhringaraj powder
  2 tablespoons Yashtimadhu powder (licorice)
  2 tablespoons Kalmegha powder
  30 drops rosemary essential oil (optional)
  30 drops lavender essential oil (optional)
  5 drops each vetiver, turmeric, and/or cilantro essential oil (optional)

1. Preheat the oven to 175°F.

2. In an oven-safe baking dish, stir the sesame oil, castor oil, Neem, Guduchi, Bhringaraj, Yashtimadhu, and Kalmegha to combine.

3. Place the baking dish, uncovered, in the oven. Heat for 8 hours, stirring every 2 to 4 hours.

4. Let the baking dish sit for 12 hours in the oven with the heat off.

5. Remove the baking dish, stir, and repeat steps 3 and 4 twice, preheating the oven again each time. This process takes 3 days total.

6. Using a fine-mesh strainer covered with muslin cloth, strain the herbs from the oil. Use your hands to squeeze out excess oil.

7. Pour the oil into a bottle or jar. Stir in the essential oils, if using.

8. Store the oil for up to 1 year.

Healthy Skin Churna

Makes 1 cup powder

Skin conditions often signify a deeper imbalance. These healthy skin herbs are cooling, bitter tonics that reduce Pitta and target the liver, two main catalysts for many skin issues. This is a tridoshic (balances all doshas) formula and beneficial for all skin types. Taking this formula daily relieves skin ailments and reveals softer, more radiant skin!

5 tablespoons Guduchi powder
3 tablespoons Bhringaraj powder
3 tablespoons Amalaki powder
3 tablespoons Manjistha powder
1 tablespoon Haridra powder (turmeric)
1 tablespoon Neem powder
2 tablespoons organic aloe vera juice (per serving; optional)
1 cup warm water (per serving)

1. In a small bowl, blend the Guduchi, Bhringaraj, Amalaki, Manjistha, Haridra, and Neem.

2. Add 1 teaspoon of herbs and 2 tablespoons of aloe vera (if using) to the water. Take upon awakening and again before bed. Be consistent for best results.

3. Store the herbs in an airtight glass jar in a dry, cool, dark environment for up to 1 year.

STRESS

Stress is the rightfully named "silent killer." Daily stressors are inevitable, but when we store stress, it becomes toxic. The first step to stress reduction is awareness. There are countless relaxation techniques, including meditation, massage, exercise, and nature walks. No matter your preference, it is essential to nourish and destress every day!

Stress Relief Tea

Makes 6 cups

Tulsi and Brahmi are magical for the mind. Ashwagandha's adaptogenic (helps body adapt to stress and encourages homeostasis) properties strengthen nerves for stress reduction. Yashtimadhu tones adrenals, and Keshar boosts mood. Enjoy this in the evenings for relief, or drink throughout the day for prevention.

4½ cups water
2 cups milk or almond milk
4 tablespoons cut-and-sifted Tulsi
3 tablespoons cut-and-sifted Ashwagandha
2 tablespoons cut-and-sifted Brahmi
7 Keshar threads (saffron)
1 tablespoon cut-and-sifted Yashtimadhu (licorice)
2 tablespoons honey

1. In a large saucepan, boil the water and milk.

2. Reduce the heat to low. Add the Tulsi, Ashwagandha, Brahmi, Keshar, and Yashtimadhu. Steep on a low simmer, mostly covered, for 20 minutes. Stir occasionally.

3. Strain and cool slightly. Stir in the honey.

4. Drink 1 cup 1 to 3 times daily for chronic stress as needed.

5. Refrigerate leftover tea for up to 5 days.

Serenity Bath Soak

Makes 3 cups

When stress is triggered, so is our sympathetic nervous system (fight-or-flight center). Warm baths are proven to invoke calmness and activate the parasympathetic nervous system (rest-and-digest center). These soothing, stress-reducing ingredients help relieve tension and relax the mind. Soak before bed for a restful sleep or any time you need a release.

4 tablespoons Shunti powder (ginger)
4 tablespoons Tulsi powder
4 tablespoons Ashwagandha powder
4 tablespoons Yashtimadhu powder (licorice)
1 cup baking soda
1 cup Epsom salt

1. In a small bowl, blend the Shunti, Tulsi, Ashwagandha, and Yashtimadhu.

2. Add the baking soda and Epsom salt. Stir evenly.

3. To use, add ½ cup to a hot bath, stirring until fully dissolved. Soak for 20 to 30 minutes. Use 1 to 3 times weekly for continued relief.

4. Store the herbs in an airtight glass jar in a dry, cool, dark environment for up to 1 year.

Tranquility Oil

Makes 4 cups

Abhyanga (oil massage) bestows a peaceful mind and strong nervous system. This oil is filled with adaptogenic (helps body adapt to stress and encourages homeostasis) nerve tonics to reduce stress and tension. Find relief through a full-body massage or a simple soothing foot rub. For severe stress, soak a cloth in the oil and place on your forehead for 20 minutes. This oil takes three days for full infusion.

5 cups sesame oil
4 tablespoons Ashwagandha powder
3 tablespoons Shankapushpi powder
3 tablespoons Brahmi powder
2 tablespoons Tulsi powder
2 tablespoons Yashtimadhu powder (licorice)
2 tablespoons Tvak powder (cinnamon)

30 drops rosemary essential oil (optional)
30 drops lavender essential oil (optional)
20 drops Tulsi or sage essential oil (optional)
5 drops vetiver essential oil (optional)

1. Preheat the oven to 175°F.

2. In an oven-safe baking dish, stir the sesame oil, Ashwagandha, Shankapushpi, Brahmi, Tulsi, Yashtimadhu, and Tvak to combine.

3. Place the baking dish, uncovered, in the oven. Heat for 8 hours, stirring every 2 to 4 hours.

4. Let the baking dish sit for 12 hours in the oven with the heat off.

5. Remove the baking dish, stir, and repeat steps 3 and 4 twice, preheating the oven again each time. This process takes 3 days total.

6. Using a fine-mesh strainer covered with muslin cloth, strain the herbs from the oil. Use your hands to squeeze out excess oil.

7. Pour the strained oil into a bottle or jar. Stir in the essential oils, if using.

8. Store for up to 1 year.

WEIGHT LOSS

Excessive weight (Staulya) is a Kapha condition characterized by too much Earth, Water, and Meda (adipose, or fat, tissue). Improper diet, emotional eating, sedentary living, hormonal imbalance, hypothyroidism, toxicity, medications, and menopause can all contribute. Obesity can create metabolic disorders and deteriorate health. Weight loss is not about extreme dieting! Adopting a balanced Kapha-reducing diet and lifestyle has proven effective for long-term results. Kindling digestion and removing toxins boosts metabolism and promotes better health.

Trikatu Tonic

Makes 1 serving

Trikatu is one of the primary formulas for Ayurvedic weight-loss programs. Its hot, penetrating nature sparks digestion, stimulates metabolism, and removes Kapha. Taking this tonic first thing in the morning awakens the vital organs and flushes the gastrointestinal tract. For simplicity, make a large batch of Trikatu (page 93) and replace the Shunti, Maricha, and Pippali with 1 teaspoon Trikatu powder.

1 cup water
½ teaspoon Shunti powder (ginger)
¼ teaspoon Maricha powder (black
    pepper)

¼ teaspoon Pippali powder
½ teaspoon apple cider vinegar
Juice of ¼ lemon
1 teaspoon honey

1. Heat the water to just below boiling and pour in a mug.

2. Stir in the Shunti, Maricha, and Pippali.

3. Cool to around 110°F and add the apple cider vinegar, lemon juice, and honey.

4. Take upon awakening. For severe weight issues, take between meals as well.

Metabo-Lite Churna

Makes 1 cup powder

This simple formula stimulates metabolism and supports digestion. Guggulu "scrapes" away fat; Punarnava balances Kapha; and Chitrak ignites Agni (digestive fire). Healthy weight is essential for optimal energy, better mood, graceful aging, and total well-being. This churna will complement any weight-loss program to support and amplify results.

6 tablespoons Guggulu powder
6 tablespoons Punarnava powder
4 tablespoons Chitrak powder
½ cup warm water (per serving)

1. In a small bowl, blend the Guggulu, Punarnava, and Chitrak.

2. Mix ½ teaspoon of herbs into the water. Take before meals 3 times daily. Be consistent for best results.

3. Store the herbs in an airtight glass jar in a dry, cool, dark environment for up to 1 year.

Agni Kvath

Makes 8 cups

Weight gain results from improper digestion. This potent decoction (kvath) will spark your Agni (digestive fire) and get things moving! This formula stimulates metabolism, flushes toxins, and removes congestion to support weight loss. Robust digestion also heightens energy, vitality, mood, and motivation!

16 cups water
8 tablespoons Punarnava powder
3 tablespoons Shunti powder (ginger)
3 teaspoons Chitrak powder
1 teaspoon freshly ground Maricha (black pepper)
6 Tvak (cinnamon) sticks
Juice of 1 lemon
½ to 1 cup honey

1. In a large saucepan over high heat, boil the water.

2. Reduce the heat to low. Stir in the Punarnava, Shunti, Chitrak, Maricha, and Tvak. Simmer, mostly covered, until 8 cups of liquid remain, about 2 to 4 hours depending on heat setting. Stir occasionally.

3. Strain using a strainer covered with muslin cloth.

4. Cool until warm; add the lemon juice and honey.

5. Take ½ to 1 cup before meals, 3 times daily. Warm with each serving, but do not heat over 110°F. Never drink cold.

6. Refrigerate leftover kvath for up to 5 days.

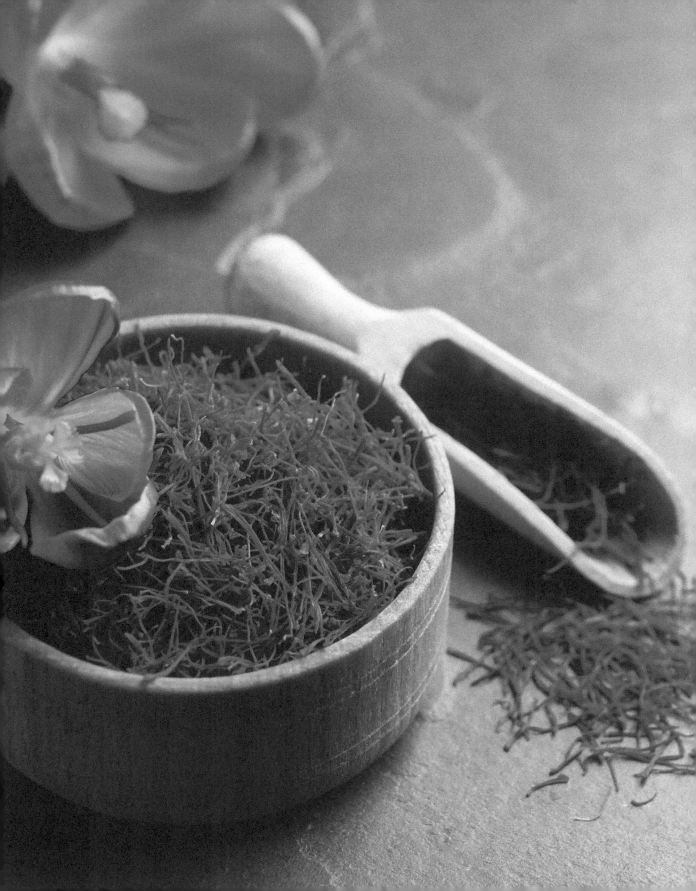

HOW TO SOURCE RARE HERBS IN THE UNITED STATES

Banyan Botanicals—Trusted organic herbal supplier. Offers rare Ayurvedic herbs, mostly in powdered form, as well as base oils. Performs third-party testing for contaminants.
BanyanBotanicals.com

Mountain Rose Herbs—Large organic supplier of high-quality Western and Eastern herbs. Offers select oils and Ayurvedic herbs and spices in powdered or cut-and-sifted form.
MountainRoseHerbs.com

Essential Organics—Provides some select Ayurvedic herbs, but many more Ayurvedic spices (powdered and whole), all organic. Offers well-priced, high-quality items.
EssentialOrganicIngredients.com

Athreya Herbs—Provides rare, organic Ayurvedic powdered herbs in bulk and offers Ayurvedic apothecary products.
AthreyaHerbs.com

Starwest Botanicals—Offers organic Eastern and Western herbs and spices in bulk, both in powdered and cut-and-sifted form.
Starwest-Botanicals.com

CITES (Convention on International Trade in Endangered Species of Wild Fauna and Flora)—Protects the interests of animals and plants in international trade. Provides a comprehensive list of endangered herbs.
CITES.org/eng

GLOSSARY

Agni: The fire element; responsible for digestion of food, thoughts, and experiences; maintaining temperature, and giving complexion and color. The main "Agni" in the body often refers to the gastric "fire."

Akasha: The ether element; provides space and freedom in our bodies and universe

Ama: A toxic, sludge-like substance that accumulates in our bodies, clogs channels, and creates disease, resulting from undigested food, emotions, and experiences

Apana Vayu: One of five subtypes of Vata; the downward-moving wind; lives in the pelvic cavity and governs defecation, urination, menstruation, and childbirth

Apas (Ap, Jala): The water element; responsible for assimilating nutrients, maintaining hydration, and providing cohesion

Artava Dhatu: Female reproductive tissue that regulates sex hormones, ovulation, sexual function, and orgasm; includes uterus, vagina, ovaries, fallopian tubes, and cervix

Asthi Dhatu: The bone tissue; provides support, shape, stability, movement, and protection; asthi indirectly relates to the hair, nails, and teeth

Ayurveda: The traditional Indian medical system, more than 5,000 years old. Comes from the Sanskrit words *Ayuh*, meaning "life," and *Veda*, meaning "knowledge" or "science."

Dhatu: The tissues forming the human body; there are seven main tissues in Ayurveda that maintain the health of the human system

Dipana: Sanskrit word meaning to "ignite fire"; a main category of herbs in Ayurveda that kindle the gastric fire (Agni) and improve digestion

Dosha: An energetic biological force that governs actions, characteristics, and dispositions; the three types are Vata, Pitta, and Kapha; the ratio in which the doshas express themselves in our bodies make up our Ayurvedic constitution, or "body type"

Kapha Dosha: The dosha made from Water and Earth; Kapha provides lubrication, support, strength, and nourishment

Majja Dhatu: The tissue of the nervous system and bone marrow; governs thought, perception, sensation, learning, and memory and produces blood cells, stem cells, and platelets

Mamsa Dhatu: The muscle tissue; provides strength, shape, protection, and support to our bodies

Meda Dhatu: The adipose (fat) tissue; consists of fats, oils, and steroids; provides lubrication, energy, insulation, softness, and love

Medhya: The group of herbs in Ayurveda that calm, heal, and strengthen the nervous system; they stimulate intellect, mood, focus, and memory

Pachana: Sanskrit word meaning "to cook"; a main category of Ayurvedic herbs that cleanse the body by "burning" toxins

Pancha Mahabhutas: The five (pancha) great (maha) elements (bhutas), specifically Ether, Air, Fire, Water, and Earth, the building blocks of creation

Pitta Dosha: The dosha made from Fire and Water; plays a strong role in digestion, transformation, processing, and critical thinking

Prabhava: A specific action an herb is most noted for; often an unexplainable, unique action that goes against the logical reasoning of taste (rasa), energy (virya), and post-digestive effect (vipak)

Prana Vayu: One of five subtypes of Vata; the inward-moving wind in the body; lives in the mind and heart and governs attention, perception, thinking, and feeling

Prithvi: The earth element; considered the building block of all matter in the universe; provides grounding, relaxation, and deep sleep

Rakta Dhatu: The blood tissue (i.e., red blood cells); carries nutrients and oxygen to the tissues and waste to the excretory organs

Rasa: The specific taste and action of a substance or experience; the six tastes are sweet, sour, salty, pungent (spicy), bitter, and astringent

Rasa Dhatu: The plasma and lymphatic tissue; responsible for bringing nutrition to the tissue and maintaining immunity, softness, and hydration

Rasayana: The classification of an herb or therapy that nourishes, builds tissues, and supports rejuvenation

Samana Vayu: One of five subtypes of Vata; lives in the small intestine and navel center; plays a major role in digestion, absorption, and assimilation

Shukra Dhatu: The male reproductive tissue that regulates sex hormones, sexual function, and orgasm; includes the penis, testicles, scrotum, vas deferens, prostate, and urethra

Srotas: A channel or pathway in the body that may be gross (physical) or subtle (energetic); there are countless channels, but 14 to 16 are the most vital

Udana Vayu: One of five subtypes of Vata; upward-moving wind that lives in the diaphragm and throat; governs exhalation, speech, memory, and enthusiasm

Vata Dosha: The dosha made from Air and Ether; Vata governs movement, circulation, respiration, sensation, and perception

Vayu: The wind element; governs all movement in living beings and in the universe; creates action, adaptability, and energy

Vipaka: The effect an herb or substance has after it has been digested; takes place in the colon and directly affects the excreta and tissues (dhatus)

Virya: The heating or cooling energy an herb or substance produces once it hits the stomach; has a direct effect on the Agni (digestion)

Vyana Vayu: One of five subtypes of Vata; lives in the heart and circulates through the bloodstream; responsible for circulation, heart functioning, and delivering nutrients and oxygen to the tissues (dhatus)

RESOURCES

WEBSITES

Alandi Ashram
AlandiAshram.org
Website of Ayurvedic school and clinic; includes blog and recipes

Consumer Version of the Natural Medicines Comprehensive Database
NaturalDatabaseConsumer.TherapeuticResearch.com
A free (but limited) online source for basic drug-herb interactions with commonly known herbs

Dr. Claudia Welch
DrClaudiaWelch.com
Website of Dr. Welch, an Ayurvedic practitioner, speaker, and author. Includes online courses and Ayurvedic articles (with hints of Traditional Chinese Medicine)

Dr. Robert Svoboda
DrSvoboda.com
Website of Dr. Svoboda, a licensed Ayurvedic practitioner and author. Includes Ayurvedic articles (with hints of Hinduism, Tantra, and Jyotish)

Drug-Herb Interaction Websites
NaturalMedicines.TherapeuticResearch.com
A very thorough, subscription-based database for drug-herb interactions

Svastha Ayurveda
SvasthaAyurveda.com
Ayurvedic blog and recipes

BOOKS

Ayurveda Beginner's Guide by Susan Weis-Bolen
A basic introduction to Ayurveda suitable for beginners who are looking to explore the foundational principles in a robust yet accessible way.

Ayurveda Cooking for Beginners by Laura Plumb
With Ayurvedic recipes, seasonal offerings, and meal plans, this cookbook will help you to incorporate Ayurvedic cooking into your daily eating.

Modern Ayurveda: Rituals, Remedies, and Recipes for Balance by Ali Kramer
Featuring a 7-day kickstart plan and Ayurvedic information with a contemporary angle, this book will prove useful for those looking to integrate a modern sense of Ayurveda into their lives.

Prakriti: Your Ayurvedic Constitution by Robert Svoboda
An introduction of the three doshas and your Ayurvedic body type for beginners to intermediate.

The 30-Minute Ayurvedic Cookbook: Healing Recipes for Total Wellness by Danielle Martin
Includes simple Ayurvedic recipes for healing imbalance, both traditional and non-traditional options.

HERBALISM COURSES

Nighantu: Advanced Ayurvedic Herbal Studies
Ayurved Sadhana (Superior, Colorado; online accessible)
AyurvedSadhana.com
Taught by Dr. Bharat Vaidya

Nighantu, Botany and Phytochemistry
Alandi Ayurveda Gurukula (Boulder, Colorado; online accessible)
AlandiAshram.org
Taught by Alakananda Ma

GENERAL ONLINE COURSES

Dr. Robert Svoboda:
Full list of online courses: DrSvoboda.teachable.com/courses

Dr. Vasant Lad:
Free online lectures: Ayurveda.com/videostream
Webinars: Ayurveda.com/webinars/overview

Foundations of Ayurveda Course (taught with Dr. Claudia Welch and Dr. Robert Svoboda):
DrClaudiaWelch.com/shop/online-courses-shop/foundations-ayurveda-1
-category/foundations-ayurveda-i

SCHOOLS

Alandi Ayurveda Gurukula
Ayurveda school and clinic; Boulder, Colorado
AlandiAshram.org

Ayurved Sadhana
Ayurveda school and clinic; Superior, Colorado
AyurvedSadhana.com

The Ayurvedic Institute
Ayurveda school and clinic; Albuquerque, New Mexico
Ayurveda.com

REFERENCES

Amalraj, Augustine, and Sreeraj Gopi. "Medicinal Properties of *Terminalia Arjuna (Roxb.) Wight & Arn.*: A Review." *Journal of Traditional and Complementary Medicine* 7, no. 1 (January 2017): 65–78. doi.org/10.1016/j.jtcme.2016.02.003.

Dash, Vaidya Bhagwan. *Materia Medica of Ayurveda: Based on Madanapala's* Nighantu. New Delhi: B. Jain Publishers, 2008. First published 1991.

Dattani, Saloni, Hannah Ritchie, and Max Roser. "Mental Health." Our World in Data, April 2018. Last updated August 2021. ourworldindata.org/mental-health.

Frawley, David, and Vasant Lad. *The Yoga of Herbs: An Ayurvedic Guide to Herbal Medicine*. 2nd ed. Twin Lakes, WI: Lotus Press, 2008. First published 1986.

Lad, Vasant. *Textbook of Ayurveda*. Vol 1. Albuquerque, NM: Ayurvedic Press, 2012.

Pandey, Gyanendra. *Dravyaguna Vijnana*. 3rd ed. 3 vols. Varanasi, India: Chowkhamba Krishnadas Academy, 2005.

Pole, Sebastian. *Ayurvedic Medicine: The Principles of Traditional Practice*. Churchill Livingstone Elsevier, 2006; Reprinted 2009.

Sharma, P. V., trans. *Caraka Samhita*. Vol. 1. Varanasi, India: Chaukhambha Orientalia, 2011. First published 1981.

Vaidya, Bharat. "Nighantu: Advanced Ayurvedic Herbal Studies" course. Course notes. Ayurveda Sadhana, 2011.

INDEX

HERB INDEX

ACKNOWLEDGMENTS

I am honored to write on a topic I hold very dear to me, but without my teachers this opportunity would never have come. I am eternally grateful for Madeleine Huish, Shandor Remete, Emma Balnaves, Dr. Vasant Lad, Alakananda Ma, and Dr. Bharat Vaidya. Without their dedication, this world would not shine so bright.

ABOUT THE AUTHOR

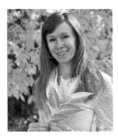

Danielle Martin is an Ayurvedic practitioner and founder of Svastha Ayurveda. She graduated from the Ayurvedic Institute and Alandi Ayurveda Gurukula. Find Danielle's writings and recipes at SvasthaAyurveda.com.

Danielle lives in Colorado with her family, Ryan, River, Starla, and Maverick. She appreciates cooking, gardening, walking, yoga, and playing silly games with her son.